CONQUER YOUR INNER DEMONS

The Ultimate Guide to Better Mental Health

Craig Marchant

Foreword by Dr John Di Battista

First published by Ultimate World Publishing 2020
Copyright © 2020 Craig Marchant

ISBN

Paperback: 978-1-922497-10-9
Ebook: 978-1-922497-11-6

Cover design: Ultimate World Publishing
Layout and typesetting: Ultimate World Publishing
Editor: Hayley Ward

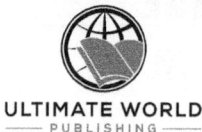

Ultimate World Publishing
Diamond Creek,
Victoria Australia 3089
www.writeabook.com.au

Dedication

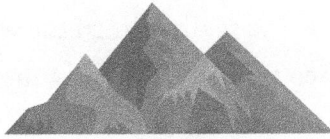

To my amazing wife Kendyl, you put up with so much – being married to somebody who has depression and schizoaffective disorder can sometimes be quite a challenge, especially as the husband enjoys stirring the pot and driving you insane.

To my beautiful children Chelsea, Jasmine, Zachery, Aidyn and Jace – you guys drive me up the wall sometimes, but I simply cannot imagine my life without all of you in it. It's not easy having a dad who is five short of a six-pack, but I hope I make up for it with lots of love.

To my mum and dad – I have a lot to thank you for in this life. You always have steered me right, even when I couldn't see it or admit it. I'm fortunate to have you both in my life, and I hope you guys hang around even longer to see what else I get up to.

To my brother and sister – wow, we sure got up to some mischief when we were younger – but I want you both to know how fortunate I feel having both of you in my life. Remember, we all make mistakes but learning from them and moving on is what it's all about!

To Cheyne, Angelo and Michael – working with you guys for all those years was an absolute blast, and I had the best time. We accomplished so much and really turned the web hosting industry in Australia on its head. Here's to many more years of success for you guys, you all deserve it.

Important note from the author

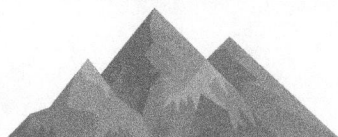

My book contains considerable information on mental health and my personal experiences with it. The advice I have given in my book is based on what has or has not worked for me, and unfortunately, mental health illnesses are different in almost every person, and so they may not work for you. My book is not intended as medical advice or to replace medical advice, and I would strongly recommend that you seek out your local health professional for a medical opinion.

It is my honest belief that you cannot do this on your own; you will need to involve health professionals to assist. Your GP/Doctor is a great place to start, and I would highly encourage fostering a partnership with your doctor and yourself. In my view, a good doctor will always listen to his or her patient and take their views and opinions into consideration, as well as their own.

Contents

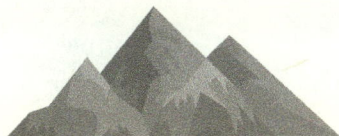

Foreword

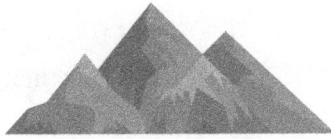

This book represents an autobiographical account of a man's journey through the inner demons of the mind. The author takes the reader through a life journey commencing with childhood, adolescence and into adulthood. He describes his transition from a regular upbringing with a supportive and loving family into a successful career in computer hardware and software development. He describes his achievements as excelling more in intellectual and business pursuits rather than physical or sporting accomplishments.

The author then poignantly describes his descent into schizoaffective disorder and the frightening world of psychosis. This occurred during his early adult years, and ultimately descended into the darkness of depression. His debilitating mental health condition went untreated in the initial years and culminated in several suicide attempts and frequent in-patient psychiatric admissions. However, the author did have one saving grace in so far as he knew that his thinking was delusional and at times was able to overcome his unreality.

After a lifetime of soul searching and fighting intermittent periods of depression and psychosis, the author undertook what could be described as a spiritual journey to identify and confront his inner demons. He reflects on his trip to the Inca Trail in 2016, where he was able to set and achieve various challenging goals, and in doing so established a new level of awareness of his true capabilities. He used this new enlightenment to re-evaluate his life and set his focus in a new life direction.

The second part of the book focuses on delivering the reader a useful and practical guide to managing mental illness based on the author's experiences in managing his own mental health challenges. It presents the reader with a detailed account of the inner workings of the mental health system, as well as alternative treatments such as medication and psychotherapy. The author also emphasises the importance of goal setting and provides suggestions to incorporate adaptive living behaviours such as sleep, hygiene, diet, and exercise. These daily living skills can improve mental health.

In my opinion, this book can be regarded as far more than a self-help book as it provides a glimpse into the personal life of an individual who has struggled to find some sense of normality within his life. He has confronted many of his life challenges head-on and has been able to achieve what could be described as an amazingly successful career. In addition, he provides the reader with a blueprint of how to successfully manage mental health problems and maintain mental stability.

I would wholeheartedly recommend this book to all readers who may have mental health issues and would like a personalised account of an individual who has successfully confronted and overcome his inner demons.

Dr. John Di Battista
Clinical & Consulting Psychologist

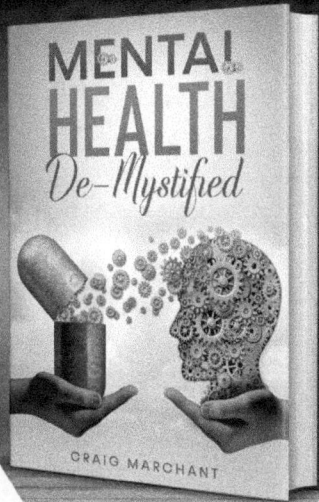

CRAIG MARCHANT

FREE eBook – Mental Health De-Mystified

Mental health issues can be difficult to recognise and can be quite challenging to bring up with a friend or loved one.

I have created this simple and easy to read resource called 'Mental Health De-Mystified' for those who have yet to be diagnosed with a mental health illness or are newly diagnosed, providing further information and practical assistance.

Go to **www.craigmarchant.com/free-ebook** to download a free copy of 'Mental Health De-Mystified'.

Introduction

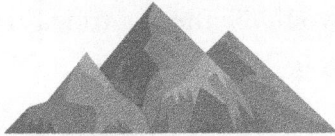

As I lay in a bed in the Intensive Care Unit of Bowral Hospital, after taking an overdose of my medication, a chance overheard conversation between another patient - an older gentleman - and the nurse would change my life for the better.

The patient told the nurse that he didn't want to die, and he wasn't ready to leave. I could hear the emotion thick in his voice and could imagine the tears that were in his eyes.

It was at that moment that I had an epiphany, my very own lightbulb moment. Here I was, in a room full of people who were desperately fighting to hold onto their lives, and I was the sole exception, trying to end my own life.

The flood gates opened, and I started to cry, weeping not only for the older gentleman but also for myself. How had my life gotten so off track? How was it that I thought the only way out of my perpetual sadness and misery was to take my own life?

Those who knew me well would have been shocked to see that I was so unhappy deep down. You see, I had perfected over many years the ability to show one thing but feel another. It was my safety mechanism. It prevented others from knowing the truth and asking questions that I was not ready to answer.

I resolved that this would be the last time I tried to take my own life and that I would get on with living my life.

PART 1

The Beginning of the Journey

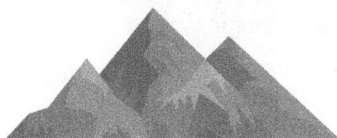

This first part of my book recounts my personal story, my journey from the start to the present day. I want to make sure you are aware, my journey includes mental health topics such as suicide, depression and schizoaffective disorder.

If you are in the middle of a mental health crisis, and by that I mean you are not stable in your illness, then it might be best to skip this first part of the book and move onto the next part. You can always come back and read this part later on when you're feeling better. Remember, my aim is to help you feel better, not drag you further into the pit of despair.

My intention for this part of the book is two-fold. Firstly, I want you to be able to see how the events of the past have helped shape me into the person I am today. Secondly, I want you to take away from my story the fact that it doesn't matter what mental health conditions you may have, you can rise above them.

Conquer Your Inner Demons!

We begin, as all good stories do, at my birth.

CHAPTER 1

My Formative Years

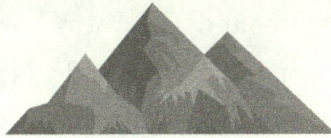

"Everyone thinks you make mistakes when you're young. But I don't think we make any fewer when we're grown up."

– Jodi Picoult

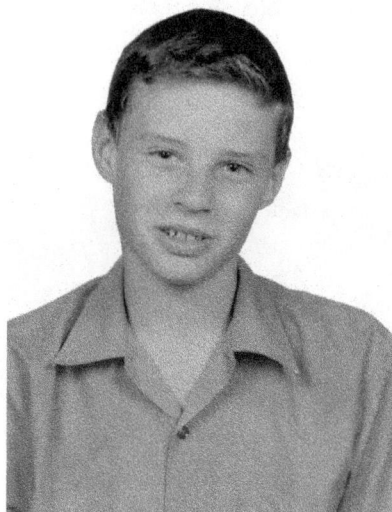

My name is Craig Marchant, and I was born on the 21st June 1981 in the Mater Hospital in Newcastle, NSW, Australia. I am the eldest child in our family, also having a younger brother and younger sister. Mum and Dad are still together, so I think myself very fortunate to have grown up with such a strong support base.

When I came along, we were living in Strathmore Road, Mallabula. I don't have many memories from there, although I do recall my bedroom. I don't remember this, but Mum tells me that as a youngster, I used to get all of my dad's plumbing pipes, etc. and build elaborate water systems in the backyard. That doesn't surprise me, as I seem to have an affinity to water, enjoying water activities such as boating, swimming, etc.

Just recently, my mum related a story to me about when I was a baby, only six months old. I had terrible eczema, so much so that even just bending a leg or arm would make the skin crack and bleed. So, the doctors put me on a combination of Phenergan and Vallergan to help me out. Mum said I was on elephant-sized doses of both medications.

Mum would also have to wrap my ankles every night. The whole procedure would entail putting a layer of moisturiser on my ankles, followed by cortisone cream. She would then wrap Glad Wrap around my ankles, followed by a bandage over the whole thing. It used to drive me up the wall. The itch was insane.

When I was around four years old, the doctors told Mum my short-term memory was abysmal and that it would plague me for all of my life. Even to this day, my short-term memory can be somewhat problematic as I can forget even mid-sentence what I'm trying to say.

Of course, Mum being Mum decided that she would show the doctors they were wrong. One time Mum told me repeatedly that she needed a few things from the shops (bread, eggs and milk). She did this for a few hours. Then she sent me into our local corner store to get those things. I came back out with two of the three things, so she counted that as a win.

Growing up in a semi-rural area, corner stores were all the rage, and we had one just down the road from us. This was before the dominance of the big supermarkets. For those who are not aware of what a corner store is, think of it like a very early version of 7-Eleven where they had the staples and often lollies, drinks, etc.

Back in the early '90s, Mum and Dad built our house at Rigney Road, Tanilba Bay. It was about five minutes away from our old house. This was to become our new family home. I spent many an afternoon swimming in our pool in the backyard. Friends would often come over to cool down on those sweltering days.

I was also somewhat active in sport and played soccer for our local soccer team as well as Little Athletics at the oval in Mallabula. I enjoyed Little Athletics and was rather good at hurdles and discus. Soccer I enjoyed also, but to be perfectly honest, I didn't think I was that good at it.

My maternal grandmother and grandfather lived down by the waterfront in Tanilba Bay, affectionately called "The Shack" a carry-over from the old house that was a shack before being knocked down and the new place built. I remember the front door for the old home was at the side, roughly where the dining room is now.

Grandfather also had a block of land in Salt Ash, NSW, which was about ten minutes away by car. He had a green thumb, and a large portion of the block was devoted to a massive vegetable and fruit garden.

My paternal grandmother and grandfather lived up the road in Tanilba Bay as well. Pa, as he was called, loved gardening and had a huge backyard which was mostly devoted to his vegetable and fruit garden. It was massive! Us kids would take turns every now and then to stay with Nan and Pa for the night even though it was only just up the road.

This part of my life I enjoyed very much.

I fondly remember my grandfather coming through the back gate to our house, and one of the first things I would hear is "G'day Dawg, what are you doing?" He was referring to one of our dogs, Pipster.

Pippy would also do his "little dance" for us. He had bad eczema and would jump up on the chairs of the outside table, reverse around and start rubbing his back against the table, making it squeak. The poor little guy would do it until he bled, although Mum and Dad would always make sure he had his cream on to try and make it better for him. I could relate; eczema is the worst.

He lived for ages; I think he was still around when I was 18, and we had him for a long time by that stage.

We had several family pets over the years. I don't remember this one, but we had a cat Dad had named "Richard the Sucker". He was a slightly confused male cat, shall we say! We had another cat that decided to move to our next-door neighbours at the time. He wouldn't even look at us when we walked or drove by. He was super spoiled, so I get why he bailed on us.

Our final cat was named Candy. Such a lovely cat, she put up with hell from us kids in the younger years.

We had a couple more dogs over the years, including a little Jack Russell who we called Patches. His other nickname was Jacque

Pierre, The Frenchman. Around the same time, my brother decided he wanted to get a dog, a gorgeous Staffy cross named Budrick. She was a big girl, but very affectionate. Her nickname was the bearded lady.

Dad loved to give the pets inventive and creative names and even talk for them, a tradition which I have continued with, as you'll learn later. Hmmm, upon reflection, maybe I never had much chance of being "normal". But you know, I would not change it for the world. I am happy being me.

Another fond memory was of our next-door neighbours Allen and Irene. They were an older couple who had a huge Ridgeback dog named Earl. We used to call him Earl the Girl. I can't tell you how lovely they both were, and they put up with us kids often. They never did complain about us kids. Upon reflection, they must have been saints :)

For primary school (Grades Kinder thru Six), I attended Tanilba Bay Public School. It was only a short walk/bike ride from our family home to the school, so that made it simple to get to school. All we had to worry about was swooping magpies in the spring. That used to get my goat; I was never attacking them, so why attack me?

We always enjoyed Christmas. Usually, I would end up helping Grandma put her tree up and decorating her house - she liked that sort of thing. It would literally take hours to put it all up. But it was nice to be able to spend time with her like that.

Then on Boxing Day, we had a big family get-together at Grandma and Grandpa's place, which was right on the waterfront. We had aunties, uncles, cousins, etc. It was a big event, and we got to spend time chatting with everyone. We usually would have about 30+ people attending. It was a good excuse for everybody to get together. I remember the blokes all watching on TV the start of the Sydney to Hobart yacht race and alternating with the cricket. Not exactly my cuppa tea, but hey.

My brother and I got up to some mischief in our time down at Grandma and Grandpas. One time, which I partly recall and partly as told by Grandma later on down the track, my brother and I were playing with my grandfather's air rifle, which we had found somehow. We were loading nails into the barrel and then firing them at the garage roller door. I'm assuming I would have been the ringleader since I was the older one. Reasonably dangerous in reflection; however, we didn't think about it at the time.

Anyway, Grandpa came to investigate what the heck the noise was coming from outside, and he found us with the air rifle. We took off at this point, running around the house. He finally caught up to us, and we copped a few smacks on the backside (rightfully so might I say)!

I found out later that as Grandpa was chasing us around the house, Grandma came out and said: "Ivan, you silly old fool, stop, and they will come to you!" And sure enough, she was right, because we did run into him.

We also used to go yabby hunting on the waterfront. When the tide was low, it uncovered a whole patch of seagrass, and we would use the yabby pump to suck them up and collect them. You could use them for fishing, etc. Half the time, it was fun just to collect them and put them in the bucket, and we would just let them go when we were finished.

I was 12 when we lost my maternal grandfather. He must have been feeling a bit off, so went for a sleep. He didn't wake up; he had a massive heart attack and died in his sleep. Reflecting on it, if you have to go, there are probably a whole lot of worse ways you can go.

I remember only a few things from that day, one was seeing him in bed (seemingly asleep), but he was ice cold to touch and very stiff. I also acutely remember my mum's distressed cries as she arrived at Grandma and Grandpa's house as she got out of the car. But most of all, I harboured much ill will towards myself on that day.

What?! I can hear you asking the question, "Why would you think you were to blame for any of this?" You see, generally, Mum would take my sister to her ballet/dance lessons, Dad would take my brother to rugby league games, and I was a bit of a free floater. Sometimes I had soccer, or I had free time. I had the option of staying with Grandfather on this day (and it was Father's Day just to add the boot in), and for some reason, I decided I would go to the football that day with Dad.

I held myself responsible for this great tragedy. Even when our local GP told me that he had a massive heart attack and nobody could have helped him, I still didn't believe it.

If I had to select a day that was the start of my mental health issues - this would be it. It signalled the beginning of a downward spiral of events in my life that would have repercussions for many years to come. If only I knew then what I know now I wonder how different my life may have been.

I was in grade six at primary school, and slowly but surely, things started to fall apart. I recall Mum and one of the teachers talking, and he said I needed to just get over it. Of course, we now know that if it were only so simple. I still liked the teacher, he was a charming teacher, and I got on well with him.

Remember, this was a time when young children didn't get depression according to the medical specialists, so it was very rare. I spent about a week in hospital, and they did every test under the sun to try and determine what was wrong with me. They did tests for epilepsy and other disorders, but nothing came up.

I'm sure I remember my mum asking if it could be depression, but the doctors assured her there was no possible way. As you might be able to tell, I don't often trust doctors - ones I have seen for some time I do, but not just any old Joe Blow.

I often ponder on what was said and think to myself, "Just because you haven't seen it doesn't mean it's not possible!" It will be interesting in another 20 years to see what medical research will tell us.

I started my fascination with computers by dismantling Mum's first computer. It was a big beefy thing, with an 8086 CPU, 20mb hard drive (was the size of a hardcover book basically) and good old MS-DOS 4 as the operating system. When Mum found out, she almost had a heart attack. But to my credit, I did manage to put it all back together again. And bonus, it even worked!

We had Microsoft Works version 3 that ran from the large 5.25-inch disks. It was fantastic as you could do word processing, spreadsheets and a database program all built into one.

Our very first printer was a dot matrix printer with a continuous paper feeding system. My God, it used to make an almighty racket when you used it. I kind of miss the sounds of the impact of the head hitting the paper. But not too much!

We would often go out boating as Dad and my uncle owned a boat together. We went out through the heads of Port Stephens to Broughton Island one time. We anchored the boat out in deep water and then swam ashore and generally had a great time. We also went snorkelling, and a dopey leatherjacket fish got into somebody's wetsuit. I still have no idea how that is even possible, but there you go.

We would also take the boat up to the Myall Lakes. It is beautiful up there, and there are plenty of places to camp. I think I may have even slept on the boat - it had an undercover area at the bow with two sorts of lounges in a V shape.

We also had an inflatable tube that we would tow behind the boat and boy oh boy, could that boat move. Pulling the tube behind was heaps of fun. I think the ultimate aim of whoever was driving the boat might have been to flip that tube :) Any number of times I can remember being flung like a ragdoll off that tube and into the water. It was, however, a lot of fun.

My paternal grandfather and grandmother owned an opal mine at Lightning Ridge. I think we went up a few times over the years. It was a fair hike to get there as it basically is at the border between NSW and QLD, a seven and a half hour car ride, and for some reason, I always think of it warmly when I hear the song Young Years by the band Dragon. I think Dad may have played it a few times while we were driving up and so now it's stuck in my head. Association, weird thing, hey?

There is also a natural hot spring pool up there; it was always so warm and lovely to go swimming in.

I used to love climbing down into the opal mine and digging for opals. We found a few over the years - it was amazing to dig them out from the earth. It even had a bucket system set up so that you could put all of the dirt from digging in and it would haul it up and out of the mine.

29

Nan and Pa had a caravan on-site and also a canvas tent that extended from the side of the caravan to give more space for sleeping. I remember sitting around the campfire in the evening and early mornings just chilling out and spending quality time with everyone.

There were a whole bunch of mines in that area, so you had to be careful where you walked at night, so you didn't end up going down a hole.

There was also a pub up there - I know, go figure hey! Not that we spent much time there ourselves.

I also have fond memories of staying at Burren Junction. That was a six hour drive, and was out in the sticks, and we stayed in a cabin, for want of a better term. I can remember a wild pig being shot and eating some rabbit. If memory serves, it tasted a lot like chicken.

We went to Leyland Brothers World for one of our annual school camps one year, which included a 1/40 scale replica of Ayers Rock, now known as Uluru. It was a bush camp and was a lot of fun. I don't recall which camp it was (must have been either grade 5 or 6) and they were giving out awards for the best student, etc. Well, I won the "Casanova" award. I had no idea who Casanova was, but when I looked it up later in life, I was somewhat embarrassed. No wonder plenty of people were snickering!

During grade six, I needed to make a decision about which high school I was going to attend. There were a few choices open to me, but I finally chose Waratah Technology High School. It just seemed like the right place for me. A few other students also decided to go to Waratah Technology High School.

High school was an interesting ride, to say the least

I completed my secondary schooling at Waratah Technology High School in 1997. It has since been renamed to Callaghan College - Waratah Technology Campus.

The school was about an hour from Tanilba Bay, so we had early starts and late finishes. I would usually get up at about 6 am, be on the bus by 7 – 7.15 am, and get to school at about 8:15 - 8:30.

For the first year, we caught the worker's bus in and out from Tanilba Bay - but by the second year, we had a dedicated bus that took us to and from school.

From grade 7, I began to experience panic attacks, which would usually culminate in me collapsing or blacking out for a while. It was rather miserable, and it continued on and off over the next four years.

I remember one time; I had just gotten off the school bus at our stop and was walking home. For some reason, my anxiety was playing up something chronic that day; my heart felt like it was beating out of my chest, and I was all hot and sweaty. I was also feeling very dizzy and lightheaded. It seriously felt like I was having a heart attack. The next thing I remember is waking up on the front lawn at our house; I must have worked myself up to such a state that I collapsed there. How long I was out for, I can't say, but I'm guessing it was a couple of minutes. This is how I felt when I had a panic attack.

Everyone's anxiety/panic attacks are a little different, and almost always, you do not faint - lucky me, hey?

The number of times I ended up in the school sickbay and having them call Mum to come and get me - I couldn't honestly count, but I know it was quite a lot. She must have been well and truly over it in the end.

I do have some good/funny recollections from school.

As I mentioned, I was pretty good at computers, so I got up to a lot of shenanigans with them.

When Mum upgraded from an 8086 to an 80386 based system, we also got our first graphic user interface system, "Windows for Workgroups 3.11". Back in the day, the operating system and graphic user interface were separate items, and you purchased them separately. It was pretty advanced for the time, and I got my first taste of video games at this point. I remember Warcraft 1 and Duke Nukem but not in which order they were acquired/played.

Windows for Workgroups had support for networking in it. I liked Windows 3.11, and it was using this GUI that I first got to experience the world of Bulletin Board systems and eventually the internet.

Eventually, we upgraded our version of MS-DOS to 5.0, and that contained QBasic, which was a programming language compiler. Hence, naturally, of course, I started to tinker with QBasic and eventually ended up playing with QBasic Version 4.5 when it was released. That was indeed my first foray into programming, thanks, Uncle Bill :) There were a number of example/demonstration programs which came with QBasic including "Nibbles" and "Gorillas". Nibbles was just a simple variant of a snake program, and I liked playing it. My favourite one, however, was Gorillas. In it, you had a very simple city skyline with a gorilla at each end of the scene. Then you had to turf a banana at the opposing gorilla trying to wipe them out. If I'm being honest with myself, I think those two games are responsible for my fascination with software programming and computer games in general.

The first modem I had was a 9600 baud internal modem. God, they were a pain in the bum to set up. Back in the older days, you had to configure IRQ and DMA settings on the internal cards, and you did that with jumpers. A jumper was simply a little black square, smaller than a thumbnail, which you placed over two metal prongs sticking out from the card to complete the circuit. I tell you, hell hath no fury like an incorrectly configured pc card!

We upgraded to an external 28.8k dialup modem, which would often cause buffer overruns because the UART Chipset that controlled the serial port on the computer was only an 8250. We ended up splashing out (thanks Mum) and getting a serial port card which had a 16550 UART Chipset (no more buffer overruns for me – YAY!).

One of my friends had a bus driver, Ross, who had a bulletin board system setup which you could dial in with your modem and exchange emails with other people - I guess you would call it the first version of email before the internet was a big thing.

The internet started to become a big thing in 1995 I believe it was, at least here in Australia anyway. Once we got the internet connected, we upgraded our modem to a 33.6k modem (which was the bee's knees at the time).

To connect to the internet, we had to use Trumpet Winsock, which was a software framework that enabled Windows-based computers to use Transmission Control Protocol/Internet Protocol (TCP-IP) features. I first used it on Windows 3.11 and then later on Windows 95.

I remember my playing around with Mum's computer landed me in some serious hot water on occasion. Another such time, I foolishly (I didn't know at the time) had replaced the Command. com binary (which was the command-line interpreter for DOS, Windows 95, Windows 98 and Windows ME) with a different version.

By the way, I had cute little nicknames for some of the windows versions. Windows NT was named "Nice Try," Windows ME was short for "Many Errors," and Windows SE was short for "Shithouse Edition".

Anyway, I had transferred the MS-DOS 6.22 Command.Com binary onto the hard drive containing the MS-DOS 5.0 operating system and then wondered why it wouldn't boot.

It took a little while, but in the end, I realised my mistake and grabbed the 5.0 installation disk and got the command.com file back on correctly. All was well in the world, although I was in some serious trouble for a while after that.

Our school had a few different networks set up; there was a Mac and a PC room. All of them were connected by what would now be considered an ancient method called Coaxial Cable. This involved a T Junction on each network card in the PC and using terminators at the end PCs.

We were using Novell Netware as the Network Operating System on the PC Network, and on the Mac's as well, I think.

I learned how to create my own coax cables at high school and the finer points of networking. It was rather intriguing to me. The school did not teach these as such as part of the curriculum; it was our computer teacher who showed us how to do it.

The havoc you could cause simply by removing a terminator from the end of a T junction was both awe-inspiring and scary at the same time.

We used to say one of the teachers could launch NASA rockets out of the school - where her office was had a pointy sort of turret and one of those ancient school roofs, like out of Harry Potter if I'm honest. And she had several computers in her office. I think I may have been slightly jealous!

One of the more "amusing" events was a bit awful to one of my friends - now that I think about it, I feel kind of ashamed of being such a bugger to him. Wherever you are Luke, lots of love mate and no hard feelings, I hope.

Anyway, Luke had snow-white hair, so naturally, we called him Snowy.

An accidental find I made early on in my computer career, was that if I modified one of the games called Space Invaders by altering a single character, it would turn into a reboot script. Now I think about it; it was probably some sort of buffer overrun or memory overrun which would, in turn, reboot the PC.

We were also learning to program at school at this time. So I wrote a program which would log in, ping every PC in the room with a rather colourful sentence, "Snowy is a fag," log back out and then execute a clean-up script to get rid of any evidence, and finally run the Space Invaders executable to reboot the

PC. It also was set on a timer, so I was not in the room when it happened.

Suffice to say, I started the program and conveniently left to go to the toilet. I didn't go to the bathroom, I just hung around outside the front of the classroom waiting for the impending mayhem to start. The program did everything as it was designed to, and no trace was left. When I returned, the teacher pulled me aside saying she could not prove it, but she knew it was me. Hey, I was bored out of my skull - which is how I justify it.

I was good at computers, but what I enjoyed even maybe more than computers was Ancient History. I was fascinated by Ancient History - and to this day, it still drives me. I want to check out Egypt and the Pyramids at one point in my life before I get much older.

We loved to fear the teacher who taught that subject. She was the type of lady who commanded respect, and you dare not put a foot wrong lest you end up on the bad side of her.

Another subject I enjoyed was Design and Technology. I remember an exchange between our teacher and two of my classmates on a fateful day.

One of the boys called one of the girls a slut, and she, in turn, called him a dickhead. The teacher had both of them stand up and then proceeded to break apart the boy calling the girl a slut, and then vice versa for the girl calling him a dickhead.

Both of their faces were red by the time this was all completed. I had a newfound respect for the teacher that day.

I played water polo for school during the warmer months of the year. I enjoy playing, but I wasn't very good at it. For school sports, we could choose from several different external activities such as ten pin bowling and lawn bowls. My friends and I would alternate between doing lawn bowls for one term and then swap to ten pin bowling for the other.

The library was my refuge at school, and I spent a lot of time there. I was a library monitor with a few other boys, so it was a slightly clicky group, shall we say. There was our librarian, the librarian assistant, and in the photocopying room, there was another assistant.

This also helped to cement my love for books. I'm particularly a fan of fantasy novels. I also rate horror highly. My favourite authors are Stephen King and David Eddings.

We used to get away with probably more than we should have in the library. We were able to use the audio/visual rooms to watch movies on VHS cassettes. This was in between operating the computers to loan out books, etc.

I recall any number of times the older kids used to cause havoc by removing the magnetic strips from library books and sticking them inside their school bags. The victim would then unknowingly walk through the detector, setting it off and causing a general commotion.

I had a few close friends in high school; some I have kept in touch with over the years and some I haven't.

I spent a lot of time with one of my friends, Nathaniel. He lived just up from school, so it was easy to walk to his place and spend some time there. His mum and dad were very lovely people, and we would play on computers or listen to music. We even went to some movie marathons at the movies at Glendale. It was three movies back to back – I really enjoyed doing that sort of stuff. Movies were a great way to escape.

These memories are some of my fondest at high school.

During this time in high school, I was also running my own computer hardware business, buying parts from OBM Computers in Cardiff and making computers for friends and family. It just felt natural to me. I guess this is where my strong entrepreneurial streak started.

The family went on an overseas trip to the USA in 1995, where we got to visit many places, including Los Angeles, Las Vegas, Grand Canyon, etc. It was a rather eventful time. At one point our car broke down, and we had to wait in a tiny little country town for the car to get fixed before we could get back on with the trip.

We also went to Disneyland and Universal Studios. I am affectionately known as the "Woosy Brother" because I'm not big on rides, so I would often sit out rides that I had zero interest in. I think Dad got me onto Matterhorn Mountain; never again thank you very much. If it goes really fast, turns upside down or anything of that nature, you can forget it thanks. I'm not called the "Woosy Brother" for no reason ☺

I remember hearing on the radio that OJ Simpson had been found not guilty, which by all accounts means we were over in the States for a couple of weeks either side of the 3rd October 1995.

This was well before the tragic events of 9/11, so security was far laxer at the airports. I wouldn't say it was terrible, but certainly, nothing like it is now.

As you can tell by now, I was an overachiever when it came to computers and the internet. I mentioned previously that our school was using Novell Netware 4 as the network operating system (NOS). This was before networking support was inbuilt into Microsoft Windows by default, so you had to rely on external software to provide the networking assistance. I was so fascinated with it that I wanted to become a Certified Novell Administrator (CNA). Mum and Dad brought me a CBT (Computer Based Training) program that I think came from a company called Educom. It came on about ten or so CDROM discs and could be run on your computer so you could learn at your own pace. After the learning, you went into a special testing centre to undertake the actual test. Conveniently, there was one located in Newcastle, so that made things a lot easier. I took the test and passed, becoming a Certified Novell Administrator, which from what I was told was no mean feat and certainly not at my age. I was pretty happy with myself, and it helped to cement the notion that if I put my mind to it, I could do pretty much anything.

I also was fascinated with fibre optics, as it was an emerging technology around that time. I think it had been around for a while but was just starting to gain major acceptance. There was a one-day training seminar on fibre optics which dealt with how to properly splice cables, and the technology behind it, etc. Naturally, I wanted to attend. Once again, Mum and Dad shelled out the money for me to attend. I can't remember if it was held in Newcastle or Sydney, but I did find it very enjoyable and certainly learned a lot that day. I even was able to splice my own Fibre Optic cables together.

There were a few negatives at high school, and one of them was my fault.

I was on my way home, and I was coming down from level one of the school via the stairs to the ground level. My big fat foot didn't fit on the stairs properly so that should have been my first sign not to be going so fast.

But I continued at breakneck speed and twisted my right ankle rather severely. It was a significant sprain; I tore some ligaments and cracked the growth plate on my ankle. It was never really right after that. I remember it swelling up massively and hobbling into one of the teacher's offices for help.

I ended up going to the hospital to have a scan done on it, and at the time, nothing was noticed being wrong other than the usual garden variety sprained ankle. However, when it was reviewed by a specialist later on down the track, he said that I had damaged some of my ligaments and had cracked the growth plate as well.

Outside of school, I used to volunteer with the Australian Coast Guard. As mentioned previously, we lived very close to the water, and this started my education on boating and operating the radios. When I got a bit older, I even used to operate the radios on my own. I had to get a special license from ACMA to be able to operate the radios. I also obtained my boating license from the Waterways Authority in NSW while I was volunteering.

One of my good friends was a guy called Richard. I used to spend lots of time with him going to computer meet and greets or other Coast Guard installations around Newcastle/Port Stephens and the Central Coast. While he was older than me, I had an absolute ball with him, and I look back at those times with fond memories. He was also a computer buff like me, so that also further cemented our friendship. We used to go to computer markets looking for all the latest and greatest stuff.

We also had a smaller boat that we kept at Grandma's - "The Tinny" as it was affectionately known. It had a smaller sized motor on it, and my brother and I used it all the time. There is a small island out in the middle of the bay where we lived called Snapper Island or as we called it, "Billy Goat Island".

We went camping once or twice on the island, which was a lot of fun, and we also went exploring. The island had reasonably dense undergrowth, so the best way to explore was around the outside of it and along the rocks. There were also quite a lot of billy goats - who would have ever thought!

During the summer holidays, which runs from around the 20th of December until the end of January here in Australia, I was enrolled to learn how to scuba dive at Nelson Bay. We started with the theory on day one, which was all classroom work. Then on the second day, we went to the local pool and got acquainted with the scuba equipment and how it all worked. Then finally, on day three, we went out to the water and had a test drive. I love to scuba dive but have not done it in many years and would need a refresher course.

I was also a volunteer team manager for my dad, as he used to coach one of the local kid's teams in NRL (Football). I was in charge of managing all the player dues and recording them in the book. I enjoyed the work and used to look forward to the weekend.

I also started working casually at what was called Bi-Lo at that time. I started as a "checkout chick," but quickly progressed to an all-rounder and did stints in the deli and fruit and veg sections. I also did the evening fill.

I also really enjoyed working there and took my responsibilities seriously. It was often said that they would call me first when they needed somebody to fill in because I was so dependable.

I do recall one major boo-boo on my behalf. I was out the back operating the forklift, and I hadn't raised the roller door fully. I went to move the forklift outside and completely stuffed the roller door. I was freaking out, but I did the right thing and called the supervisors. I don't recall what the outcome was, but I can assure you I never made that mistake again!

"Doing all the little tricky things it takes to grow up, step by step, into an anxious and unsettling world."
– Sylvia Plath

CHAPTER 2

The Journey to Adulthood

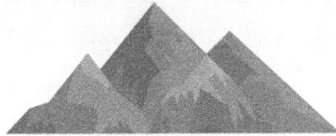

"I'm a greater believer in luck, and I find the harder
I work the more I have of it."
– Thomas Jefferson

I had decided I was going to complete Year 11/12 at high school, but over the summer holidays, I made a decision that I would do a diploma as a Programmer/Analyst at TAFE Tighes Hill Campus in NSW.

I started to do the course, but because of the damage I had done to my ankle in high school, I needed to have surgery to try and fix it. Of course, after the surgery, I had to take some time off from school to allow my foot to heal properly. It was at this unfortunate juncture that I started watching daytime soaps such as The Young and the Restless and Days of our Lives.

The only thing I can recall from this period is that a daemon had possessed Marlena in Days of our Lives. Riveting stuff, right? Worthy of being in my memory and occupying valuable space.

I ended up being off school for a month or two, and when I returned, I realised it was going to be very difficult to catch up to everyone else. I did try for a few days, but in the end, I realised it was a pointless exercise and so made the decision to finish up with the course.

Right at this point, is when I first started to experience my schizophrenic symptoms. They were really mild and quite infrequent, so, to be honest, I didn't pay them as much attention as I should have. If I could go back and do it all again, I would go and see a psychiatrist well before I did.

It wasn't anything too far out there that I was experiencing - the occasional vision and voices that were telling me I wasn't worth it, and I should just kill myself and be done with it all.

I just ignored it and kept on going.

I decided to hit the workforce and started as a hardware technician for a local computer hardware company in Newcastle called QFlow. I spent about a year there, helping to build and install PCs. I rather enjoyed it and got some valuable network and programming experience under my belt as well.

We would have competitions on who could build a computer from scratch the quickest. All the components would be in the one spot, and you just assembled it and got Windows installed as quickly as possible.

I wrote an online quoting program that ran on an Access Database and used Visual Basic. I also set up a Cisco 1600 series router to connect to the internet for the shop.

Above our shop, we had a local internet service provider called Hunterlink, which funnily enough was my ISP (Internet Service Provider) before I even started working for QFlow. It was great being able to talk to the guys, and I got to see their hardware setup, which was pretty cool. I still remember to this very day their two name servers (DNS) which were set up on two Alpha Sparc servers, if memory serves.

alphaa.hunterlink.net.au - 203.12.144.6
alphab.hunterlink.net.au - 203.12.144.7

Hunterlink even powered our internet connection in the shop. Because we were below them, they simply dropped a serial cable down into our offices, and we used that to connect to the internet. It was cutting-edge stuff at the time!

I used to make runs from Newcastle to Five Dock in Sydney to pick up computer hardware we needed for the shop in Newcastle. I wasn't a big fan of driving in Sydney, and to this day, I still am not a major fan, but I always did it.

I was then poached by another company called QPoint Australia.

QPoint was a client of QFlow - and they asked me if I would like to join up with them. They wanted to start an Amazon like-store experience, but we never could crack the market. It wasn't for lack of trying, that's for sure. We tried our hardest to get it all going, but sadly it wasn't to be. This was in the age of the dot-com bubble, which went from roughly 1994 to 2000.

It was during this tenure that we had to deal with the "dreaded" Y2K bug. It was going to be the end of the world as we knew it, but in reality it was kind of lacklustre and wasn't much to write home about from my perspective.

I do remember I learned a lot from a few of the guys there, James and Stephen. James lived life as he wanted, and I admired that a lot. He was very approachable and was always happy to sit down and have a chat. If I was ever to see him again, the first thing I would say is thank you for helping me cement my love for business again.

I moved to Bowral, NSW in the Southern Highlands and was working as a systems administrator for one of the local ISPs in town called Ace Internet Services. It was fascinating for me, as I love the internet, and here I could mix both the internet and Linux in one environment.

Unfortunately for me, my schizoaffective disorder started to play up more and was causing me some issues. Still, I just kept my mouth shut and kept on plugging away reasoning that eventually it would go away (if only I should be so lucky).

I wasn't much of a social person, so I tended just to stay home where possible and avoid people. I only lasted six months, before I found loneliness and isolation to be too much to bear, so I moved back to Newcastle.

Take note that I hadn't done much to help myself at this stage, so I had undiagnosed mental health issues I was experiencing daily.

I worked for another local company in Newcastle for about 12 months, when I happened to reach out to one of the team at Ace in Bowral saying how much I missed working there.

Lo and behold I received a phone call saying if I wanted to come back, they would more than welcome me back into the fold. After weighing the pros and cons of the situation, I decided to head back to the Southern Highlands and take up my original position again.

It was around this time that my depression was in full swing, and then I was diagnosed with schizoaffective disorder. I always recounted it like a horror movie being played, but instead of being the audience, you were the lead role, and it was being played out from your eyes instead of you watching it.

Some of it was just plain scary, I'll be honest. But I was blessed that I could usually tell what I was seeing was bullshit. That's a pretty remarkable thing from what I've been told, since often, you cannot tell.

Unfortunately for me, the wheels fell off in 2002 and after managing to keep everything together for so long, it finally all went to pieces on me. It was the start of a treacherous few years, frequent suicide attempts and hospitalisation. I think we were on a first-name basis at the hospital for quite a while.

I would work myself up into such a state that I wouldn't be thinking clearly anymore and would swallow any medication I could find. After 10 to 15 minutes, my sanity would return, and I would be left with the awful realisation of what had just happened again. What followed was the necessary phone call to emergency services and being transported to hospital for treatment.

By the way, the treatment for swallowing a lot of medicines is liquid charcoal, and it truly is the foulest of all creations. It does its job, however, which is to absorb excess medications in your stomach.

I was continually seeing my GP at the time, and my treating Psychiatrist. Between them and the hospital there, I managed to navigate my way through this very tumultuous time of my life. You might recall from earlier that I have a distrust in doctors, so you might be wondering why I was so reliant on my GP.

On the first admission into hospital, my doctor happened to be the one that I would later call my GP and also somebody I could come to rely on. Why? On my second admission into hospital, he came to see me again and said that at first, he thought I was just attention seeking but now he could see he was wrong, and I really did need substantial help. That sort of honesty showed me that he was a person who could accept that sometimes he was wrong, and for that he had my trust.

I remember several different events from that period of my life.

I was in the hospital ward after being admitted for observation, and I was still feeling somewhat suicidal, so one of the nurses was going to have to watch me for a few hours. Anyway, just before the nurse came in, one of the managers of the hospital came through the doorway asking me what my problem was. He was pissed off about the fact that he was losing a nurse for a while and chose to take it out on me. I did tell the nurse what happened, and she was really lovely about the whole thing.

Another was being sectioned under the Mental Health Act of NSW by my psychiatrist because I had just admitted that I didn't want to be alive anymore and had a few plans just to slip away. I remember it for a few reasons.

One: I was told that under no circumstances should you ever let yourself be sectioned against your will. If you are told you need to go to a psychiatric hospital, nod and agree. Why? If you let the psychiatrist section you against your will, you lose any ability to check yourself out when you are feeling better, and that is not good. Never leave the choice in the hand of the system if you can avoid it.

Two: Being in the hospital psychiatric ward at Goulburn Hospital was a bit of an eye-opener. There were some seriously messed up people there, as you would expect. Much respect to the nurses and doctors, it can be pretty full-on.

It took several years and many psychologist/psychiatrist/doctor appointments before I finally got myself to a state that I was pretty happy with. I wasn't a bundle of joy, but I was no longer trying to hurt myself and generally was glad to be alive.

It should also be noted that I maintained full-time employment during this phase of my life. I was lucky my employer was so good to me. I indeed repaid in kind with working my tail off.

In fact, when I was bored at home and had nothing to do, instead of watching TV or a movie I would often just go into work and continue with that instead so I didn't get bored, which was quite often actually. It was a great arrangement if you ask me.

I know not everybody is like I was, but if you are suffering from depression and don't have much in the way of family around or friends - doing something like I did might be of benefit to you as well. It certainly helps keep your mind occupied.

It was in 2005 that I decided to put up a profile on one of the dating websites as I was tired of being alone and lonely. I had waited for a few years until my mental health conditions were better treated, as I had always reasoned with myself that I didn't want to subject anyone to that crap.

I met a local girl, Kim, in 2005. We got married in 2006 and subsequently got pregnant with our first child. It was quite a whirlwind romance.

We got ourselves two female cats which we named Pixie and Salem. Salem was pretty much black all over with some white patches. Pixie was brown. We then decided to get two more female cats who we named Blossom and Minka. Blossom is grey, and Minka is black and grey. And then to top it off we inherited a male kitty cat which we named Dexter, all ginger. Our little ginger ninja.

Pixie's nickname was Pixie Poodle, Salem's was Salama Berry Black or ABC (Angry Black Cat). Blossom is Blossima Berry Baby, and Minka's is Stinky Minky. Dexters was Dekektor.

It was a month or two before our wedding that I reconnected with a long-time friend from Waratah Technology High School, Cheyne. As he tells me, he used his power with one of our Telcos to look up my details and reach out.

I was thrilled to reconnect again; he was my best friend in high school before he left for Queensland early in Year 10. I often wonder if part of the reason I didn't hang around for year 11 or 12 was that he wasn't around.

We were both natural computer geeks and had been running our businesses since we were both 14.

Kim and I moved down to Berwick in the South Eastern Suburbs of Melbourne in October of 2006. The reason we moved is that Cheyne wanted me to start working with their newly-formed company, Jumba – a web hosting and domain names company. So, I finished up with Ace and headed on down.

It was tough without having any of our family around to help us, but we seemed to be doing ok.

On the 29th of November 2006, our first daughter Chelsea Rose was born at the Monash Medical Centre in Clayton, VIC.

In August of 2007, we received an offer for Jumba from another competitor who wanted to purchase us. We agreed, and I finished up working for Jumba that month.

In December of 2007, I was hired by Instra Corporation/ Domain Directors, a domain name registrar business, as their IT Manager. I had earlier successfully recovered a corrupt MySQL database for them, and so they were impressed with my skills.

On the 26th of October 2007, our second daughter Jasmine Emily was born at the Monash Medical Centre in Clayton, VIC.

In June of 2008, I finished up working with Domain Directors/ Instra Corporation and started up a new web hosting and domain names company with three of my friends. The first couple of years were brutal, to say the least. We would be working the helpdesk and system admin tasks during the day, and then at night, we would head into the datacentre to install new servers or configure network equipment.

On the 15th of January 2009, my first son, Zachery Liam, was born at the Monash Medical Centre in Clayton, VIC.

Unfortunately, during this time, I decided that five cats were just too much work, and we were having trouble looking after them all. We made the sad decision to surrender two cats to one of the local animal shelters. Pixie and Dexter were selected as the two cats to be surrendered. I still feel awful about it to this very day, but I just couldn't keep up with everything. I'm hoping they did indeed get rehomed but will never know.

We were still working our tails off in the new business, but things were looking up. In December of 2010, my first marriage hit the rocks, and it became very much apparent that it had run its course and would now end.

We both did our best to keep things civil for the sake of the kids if for no other reason. To this day I don't think there is any hatred between us; that kind of thing is counterproductive and doesn't achieve much.

It was a very emotional time for me. I moved out of the family home and got a small two-bedroom flat in Pakenham, VIC, where I lived for about six months.

At first, my eldest daughter Chelsea didn't understand. I can't say I blame her as break-ups are never easy on anyone. She kept demanding to my ex that she bring her daddy and his computers back right now.

I ended up spending a few days in Berwick Hospital in the psychiatric wing, as I was not coping at all. While I don't recall everything that was going on, I was very close to the edge again and remembering what it did to me back early on in my life; I didn't take any chances.

I got out a few days before Christmas as I was starting to feel a little better about everything.

Christmas came and went, and life continued onwards.

In March of 2011, I reached out to a beautiful young lady by the name of Kendyl on an online dating website. I wasn't expecting a reply, but one arrived back in my inbox.

We had our first date at a local restaurant in Pakenham, VIC called La Porchetta. I remember I copped a lot of flak from my mates at the time because it wasn't really what you would call a romantic date location, however, we both enjoyed ourselves, so I guess that is what counts, isn't it?

We wanted to get engaged, but first, I had to finalise my divorce paperwork with the courts before that could occur. In Victoria (and I assume most/all of the other states of Australia) you have to be legally separated for 12 months before you can file all the relevant divorce paperwork.

Since Kim and I had separated in December of 2010, we had to wait until December 2011/January 2012 before that could happen.

I remember we participated in the World's Greatest Shave for the Leukaemia Foundation here in Australia in 2013. We had decided we would get a number 1 haircut using the shavers; however, somehow, we forgot to put the number on when doing my shave - so it was indeed a complete shave, not just a partial one.

We were married on April 12, 2014, at Chateau Wyuna in a beautiful ceremony followed by our wedding reception. Chelsea, Jasmine and Zachery were involved in the wedding as flower girls and page boy. They looked so cute in their dresses and suits.

Kendyl and I had our first son Aidyn on the 31st January 2015 at Monash Medical Centre in Clayton, VIC. It was a very different experience to the first three kids because Kendyl had planned with her doctor if it looked like Aidyn was not going to budge; they would move her straight to a C-Section.

Of course, doctors being doctors (I told you I have trust issues) decided not to follow the plan that had been laid out and tried to induce Kendyl, unsuccessfully may I point out. It got to midnight on the 30th of January, and I had enough of seeing Kendyl in so much pain with absolutely zero movements from the little bugger snuggly inside and promptly delivered a serve to the doctors and told them to pull their finger out and organise the C-Section.

An hour or so later, we were in the operating theatre waiting for our baby boy to grace us with his presence. He was a big boy; I called him toddler baby and Kendyl called him Buddha baby.

I got to hold him and then heard the doctors say, "We can't stop the bleeding, get the father out please". Imagine for a moment hearing those words, then being escorted out of the theatre and sitting alone with your new baby in the hospital room, wondering if you still had a wife or were going to be raising the little one on your own.

Eventually, Kendyl arrived back in the hospital room, much to my relief. Aidyn did have to go into the Special Care Nursery because he had a lot of gunk on his lungs and was having trouble breathing. The nurses all commented on how big he was, as they were used to the preemie babies being in there.

Kendyl and I had our second son Jace on the 8th March 2017, also at Monash Medical Centre in Clayton, VIC. The same hospital delivered all five of my children. This experience was also different, but in a good way. The C-Section had been planned and was executed with near perfection.

Jace's arrival was so much easier than the first time around with Aidyn. There was none of the fanfare, and I think Kendyl got out of the hospital the very next day because she had a gutful from the first time!

At work we had an annual management retreat - sometimes it was Queensland, others it was Fiji. While it sounds like a complete holiday, we would often spend long hours going through all aspects of the business trying to find ways in which we could improve our offering. Occasionally we would go for a swim or take a break before getting back into it. So generally speaking, it was all about work, but we did mix in some pleasure

I also went to the USA several times over the years. The main reason was to attend web hosting conferences that were run by various companies/suppliers. It was a great way to strike up conversations with our suppliers and do product research. There was also our tradition to head to Orlando to visit the theme parks there. Universal Studios and Disney world are enjoyable places where we could relax.

We met our original customer service manager Brandon working at Universal Studios. We would do the VIP tour at Universal because it meant we could go straight to the front of the ride lines and get access to all sorts of backstage areas and Brandon would be our tour guide.

The business continued to grow at breakneck speed, and we relocated from my best mate's house where we all worked from the same office into our first office in Verdun Drive, Narre Warren. We were only there for around 12 to 18 months before we relocated again due to putting on so many new staff. When we moved in, there were 5 of us I believe, and when we vacated the first office, we had about 10/12 staff members.

We had also taken on several remote staff as finding a locally based team wasn't an easy task as we were about an hour from Melbourne City/CBD.

We then moved into a much larger office in Victor Crescent, Narre Warren. We had a lot of spare space so that we could expand quickly. By the end of 2015, we had about 25/30 staff members comprising technical support staff and administrators, sales staff, development staff and management.

We operated three core companies at that time. VentraIP Australia was the main company and was predominantly aimed at business customers and resellers, Zuver was aimed at budget customers, and Synergy Wholesale was our domain name registrar business and also did web hosting and domain name reselling. That was the company that held our ICANN accreditation along with auDA and many other accreditations.

> "When we strive to become better than we are, everything around us becomes better too."
> **– Paulo Coelho**

CHAPTER 3

Trekking the Inca Trail

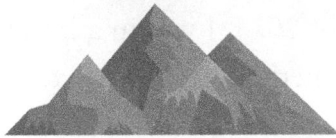

"Life comes with many challenges. The ones that should not scare us are the ones we can take on and take control of."

– Angelina Jolie

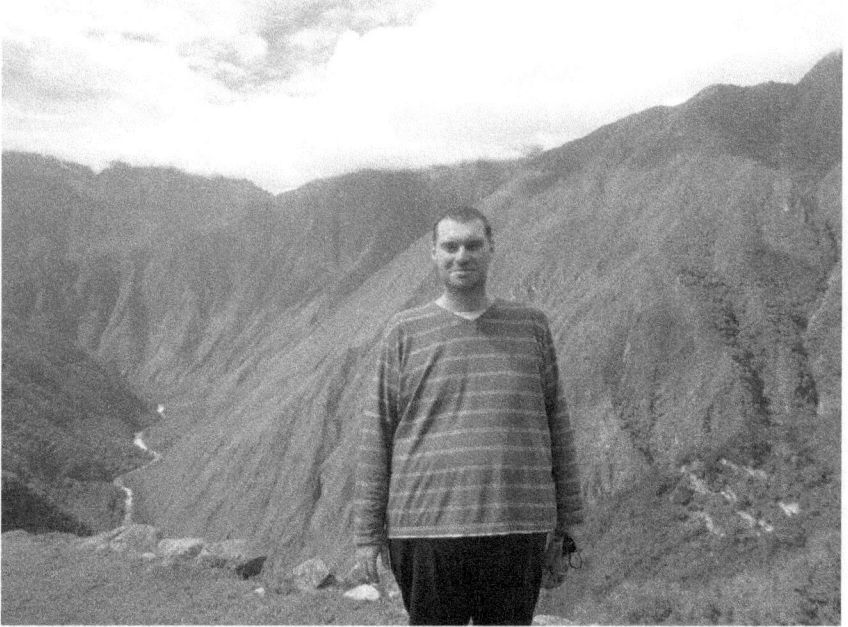

Back in November of 2015, I was in a bit of a rut at work, and I was looking for something to sink my teeth into.

I had been talking with my mum about her adventure, Plan's Cycle for Girls - a charity dedicated to improving education for girls in poorer countries. Mum said that the girls were overlooked most of the time, and only the boys received an education. I was very proud of my mum for stepping out of her comfort zone and doing something she was passionate about and believed in.

She said it opened her eyes and changed her for the better. It sounded exactly like what I needed.

I have always been passionate about helping charities; I was the team manager for my dad's rugby team when I was younger and was also a Coast Guard volunteer for several years operating the radios and going on the occasional boat outing.

Mum suggested I check out Inspired Adventures as they did a heap of adventures every year and I might find something that tickled my fancy.

Any charity there would have been a worthy option for my fundraising, but I finally settled on trekking the Inca Trail in Peru for the Leukaemia Foundation in Australia. Having helped raise funds for blood cancer research previously, it seemed like the right fit.

I should point out that I was not doing an awful lot of exercise at this time but had the gastric sleeve operation, so my weight was slowly coming off. As part of the challenge, we were also recommended an exercise guide that would help prepare us for the Inca Trail. It started slowly and then progressed to more and more exercise before backing off in the last few weeks so we wouldn't be tired for the upcoming challenge.

As part of the challenge, I needed to fundraise a minimum of $4,000 to donate to the Leukaemia Foundation. I had not had to fundraise in a long time, so this was very challenging.

I held a few different events, such as a go-karting day with my mates at work and a sausage sizzle at our local Westfield shopping centre. I even approached several different companies to sponsor me as well.

My three businesses; VentraIP Australia, Zuver and Synergy Wholesale, as well as a few other companies sponsored me, which I was very grateful for.

In the end, I managed to fundraise $5,624 for the Leukaemia Foundation, which I was pleased with.

The entire challenge was approximately 13 days in length, including flights and travelling. The Inca Trail challenge itself was five days long, and considering it was the reason I was there, I have gone into some detail about the entire journey.

Day 1

After an early start, we headed towards Ollantaytambo (2/2.5hrs travel by bus) to investigate the town and ruins located there.

After stopping to buy the last remaining items needed before starting the trek, we split up into two groups. One group looked around town and saw some of the local housing while the other group ascended the stairs of the ruins, took photos and listened to the history of the area.

Back on the bus, we headed to the start of the trek, where we had lunch and met our porters for the trek.

Let me just say in hindsight these guys are fantastic and we couldn't have done the trek without them.

They cook some real mean grub, let me tell you – in fact during the whole trek we ate fantastic food prepared by the chef and his assistant.

After a quick rundown, the porters weighed the bags (they are allowed to carry 21kg – 25kg for the company and 4kg for their items), we headed off to the checkpoint. At the checkpoint, we showed our passports and tickets and then crossed the bridge, and we were off.

It was approximately 2 pm at this stage, so we walked for three or so hours until we reached our first campsite of the trek (Llactapata).

The campground was situated 2,788m above sea level in between the valleys of Aobamba and the Salcantay.

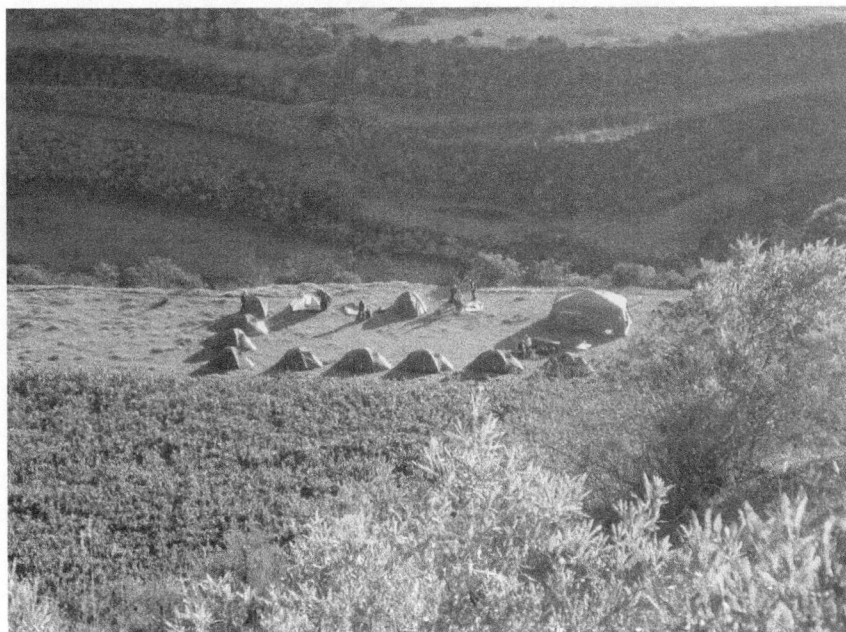

This was next to ancient ruins and a running river; very magical.

After getting settled into our sleeping tents, we had an afternoon snack and then dinner an hour and a half later.

We had our day one debriefing and day two briefing just after dinner and then took to our tents for a well-deserved rest.

Day 2

Waking up early, we had breakfast and set off on day two of the trek.

First off, we explored the ancient ruins near the campsite.

Day two was very challenging for me; I think the sheer enormity of what we were doing finally settled in, and by about midday, I was exhausted and suffering from the effects of altitude sickness. At the day two checkpoint, I almost called it quits. I simply didn't think I could do this.

Speaking with the lead guide and the other guides they said that I could turn back and meet the team in Machu Picchu, but they thought I had it in me to complete the trek. Hearing this, something inside just clicked, and that was it – my mind was made up. This wasn't going to beat me; I was going to make it all the way to the end.

We reached our campsite at around about 4:30/4:45 pm – the sunlight was just starting to retreat, and it looked amazing.

Llulluchapampa was a fantastic campsite located approximately 3,680m above sea level.

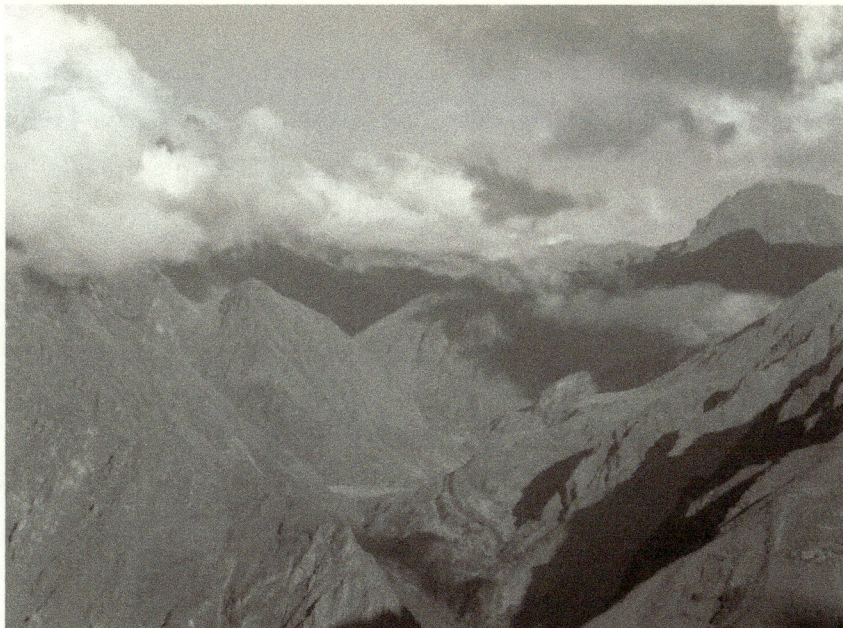

During dinner, we were asked to give some background on ourselves and what our motivations for the trek had been. Listening to all the stories the group had and the experiences with Leukemia was very humbling and altogether a rather emotional section of the night. So many brave and strong people in our group, all united by a common cause – to further Leukaemia research.

Bedtime came, it was freezing during the night, but I managed to sleep very soundly.

Day 3

On waking, we all knew it was going to be a big day for us. Today is the longest day wise as well as ascending Dead Woman's Pass, descending again and then climbing to our second peak of the day and descending.

After having our breakfast, we set off on our way. Jimmy (our lead guide) thought it best I lead the group up the pass, a two or so hours ascent of the stairs to Dead Woman's Pass. We all did amazingly well on this and getting to the top of the pass was an achievement in itself – 4,200m above sea level. What a fantastic view.

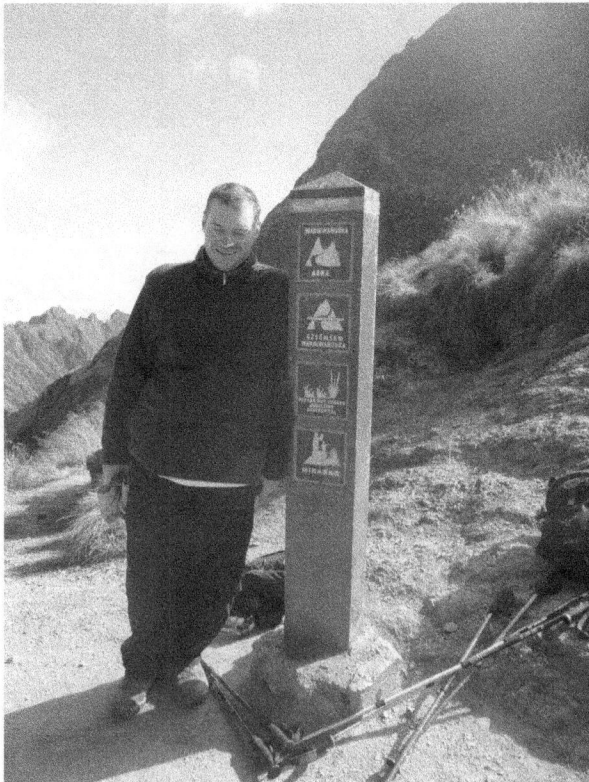

Descending the stairs into the valley below, we then started our ascension to the next peak of the day.

After stopping here for a little while, we started to go down again, noticing that the clouds were building. We were approximately 45 minutes away from our lunch spot when the heavens opened, and the deluge came down on us. It even caught the guides off guard since it usually doesn't rain in May on the trek and if it does, it's often only spot rain.

Getting to our lunch spot, we were drenched/cold, and I was feeling rather abysmal. After lunch, the rest of the group headed to the campsite under the watchful eyes of two of the guides, and the other guide and I slowly made our way to the campsite.

Suffice to say it was a very long day, and we finally made it into the campsite at 7.00 pm. After resting and getting warm we had dinner, but I didn't linger long as I was so tired. In bed, I fell asleep and slept probably the best I had on the trek.

Day 4

After a rather abysmal night, but an excellent sleep, I woke up feeling somewhat refreshed.

Our campsite, Phuyupatamarca, was located approximately 3,650m above sea level – we were camping above the clouds!

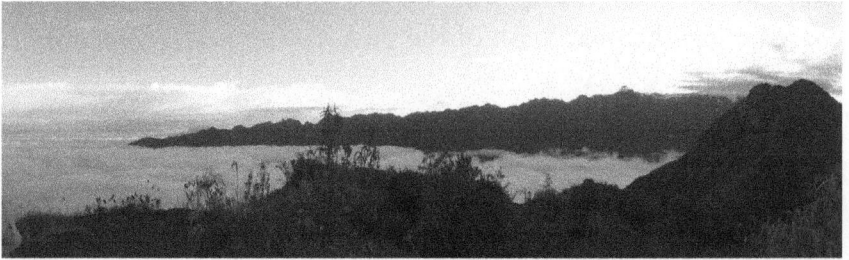

After breakfast, we set off on the final leg of our trip to the Sun Gate at Machu Picchu.

We descended from the "Place above the Clouds" and passed some ruins, as we continued onto lunch. Lunch was great, and it was there sadly, we bid farewell to our lovely team of porters who had done such an amazing job for us—what a fantastic bunch of people.

Continuing along, we got towards the "Gringo Killers" a set of stairs aptly named if you ask me as they are exceptionally steep.

After that, it was just a short hike and one last final set of stairs until we were at our final destination – The Sun Gate (Machu Picchu). What a fantastic view! It was very emotional for all the team. We had all worked so hard to get here, and finally, here it was.

After photos and relaxing for 10/15 minutes we descended to Machu Picchu and the bus stop which would take us into Machu Picchu town. We got squared away in our hotel, went upstairs to level six for pre-dinner drinks then headed off for our meal.

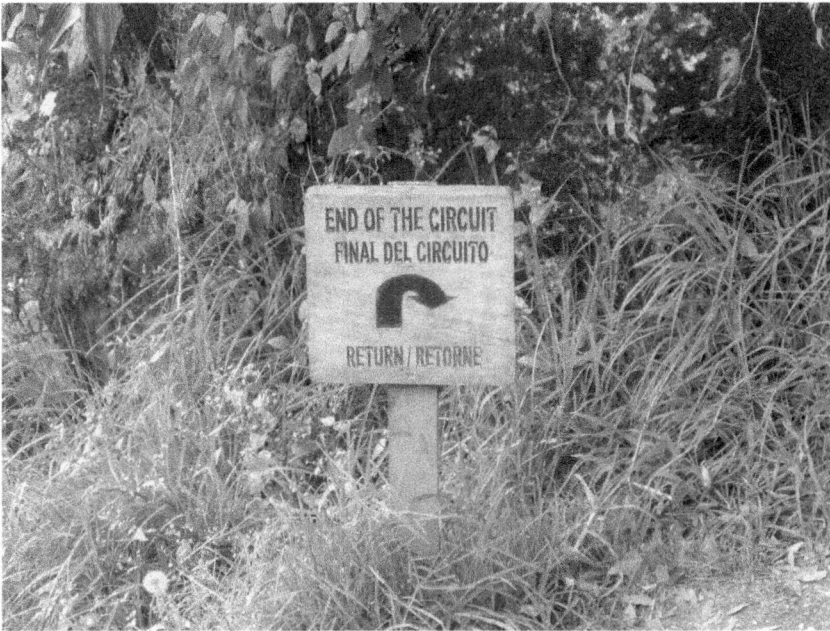

There was a religious festival on as we walked up the street, with an entire parade going down the road. I wish I had brought my camera; some of the costumes and designs were simply out of this world.

After that we headed to bed – I woke up at about 1 am and went for a little wander to have a look around and met one of the bar attendants from earlier in the evening at our hotel. He was a lovely guy and showed me around. I then headed back to the room at about 2 am and got some more sleep.

Day 5

Woke up feeling somewhat refreshed after a decent night's sleep and a hot shower.

The team made their way up from the bus stop in Machu Picchu Town (Aguas Calientes) up to Machu Picchu Ruins for our tour.

What a fantastic place, the ruins are spectacular. After much climbing and descending of stairs and taking all the photos we could, the group split up, with one group continuing the tour and then heading back to town for a well-deserved beer and the other group going up the mountain.

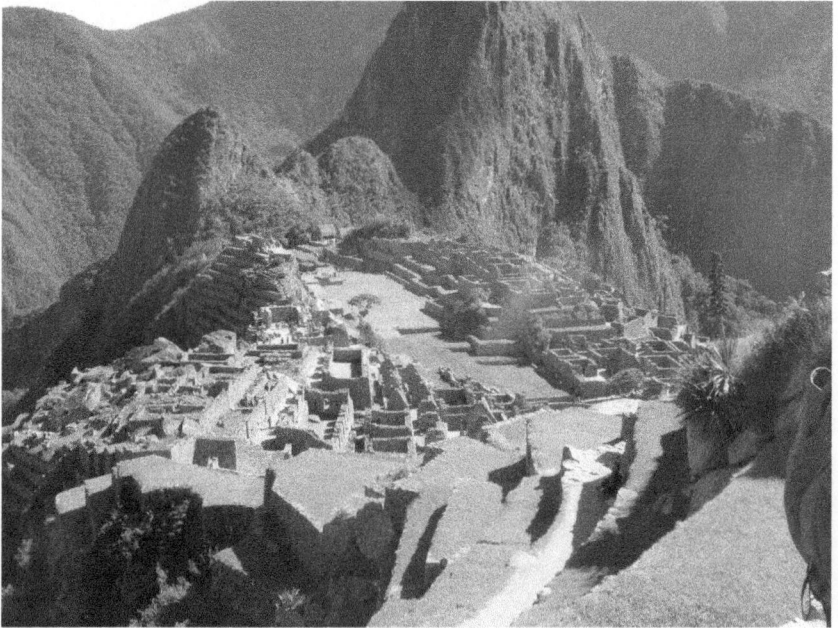

Although I did have a ticket to do the climb, there was one thing that was painfully evident to me over the last four days and that was that I'm rather slow going up, and I was also physically exhausted, so I opted not to climb it.

The group re-joined in town for lunch – a fantastic place called Indio Feliz; the food was terrific. I opted for the quiche, and the apple pie and ice-cream for dessert. Feeling full, the team left for the train station.

We hopped aboard the train headed to Ollantaytambo and settled in for a two- or so-hour train ride. We were in F Class, no idea what that means, but it was good. We got drinks and a snack and later on the staff in that carriage put on a fantastic fashion show showing off all the alpaca clothing available.

After arriving at Ollantaytambo, we headed to our bus for the two and a half-hour ride back to Cusco. Back in Cusco, we headed to our rooms to settle in. What a fantastic day.

When we got back to our rooms, I was sitting on the steps outside of my room, and our team leader approached me. He asked if I ok, and I said I felt a little bit down actually.

He said it happens to him as well, and he suggested it was because I had been working towards this goal for the better part of six months and finally it had been achieved, and I was left wondering, what's next for me?

I was surprised at how well that describes me now, and the more I thought about it, the more I was sure that was what was going on for me as well. I arrived home, my wife tells me I looked half-dead, but I think it was just from the sheer exhaustion of the trek and the associated travel back home.

"We proved that we are still a people capable of doing big things and tackling our biggest challenges."
– Barack Obama

CHAPTER 4

My Higher Calling

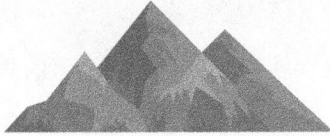

"Everyone has challenges and lessons to learn –
we wouldn't be who we are without them."
– Sean Combs

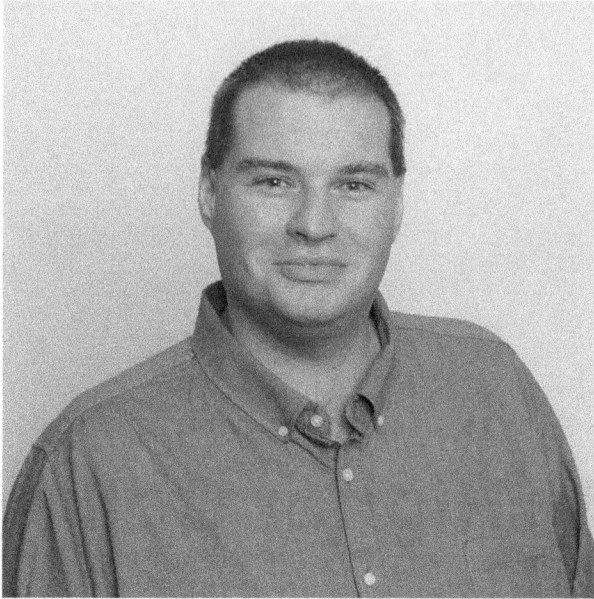

After a few days of rest, I went back to work, but I must be honest, I felt a big disconnect between myself and the businesses. I kept thinking to myself, is this all there is, is this my real purpose in life?

At first, I thought it was just because my depression was playing up with the end of the trek, but it continued to be a recurring theme over the next few months.

What I wanted to do was help people achieve their goals and navigate their way through their mental illness successfully. I wanted people to be able to look at my life story and to think to themselves, hey if he did it, why can't I?

So, I finished up with VentraIP in September of 2017. I had mixed emotions around that time. I was excited to be starting a new chapter of my life but was also sad at leaving the businesses I helped build over the years and all the friendships I had built up.

I had a few software projects that clients had asked me to do for them, which has kept me pretty busy over the last few years since I left VentraIP. I've enjoyed the variety of the work and have several contacts who often reach out for the occasional hour or two of work.

But where I've spent a reasonable amount of time has been on my professional speaking about my mental health challenges and how the Inca Trail helped me to realise what I wanted to be doing.

In February of 2019, I attended the Speakers Institute Premiere Bootcamp, which ran from the 22nd February until the 24th of February in Sydney, NSW.

I had seen the owner of Speakers Institute, Sam Cawthorn up on stage a few times before. The first was at the Capital Pitch Entrepreneurs Conference held in Melbourne on the 13th October 2017, and his story was mesmerising.

On the 10th February 2018, I attended The Mastering Storyshowing for Influence and Authority day event, which was even more tantalising seeing and hearing more of Sam's fantastic story.

I left from this event knowing that I wanted to take up the Premiere Bootcamp, however, it would take another year before that was going to happen. But I still didn't have a clear-cut path as to what I wanted actually to achieve.

What was I passionate about that I could get up on stage and deliver with certainty and conviction?

I had a few choices open to me. Computers and information technology was one area I was passionate about, especially with regards to the Internet.

I was also an expert on my own depression and schizoaffective disorder, and maybe just maybe my story might be the encouragement that somebody out there needed to continue fighting the good fight and getting the help they needed.

On day one of the bootcamp, I got to the venue about 20 minutes late due to my scheduled flight being cancelled and having to get a different one and then the famous Sydney traffic.

I slunk my way into the room and was given all the information needed. People were up on stage already, with a getting to know you session. You needed to speak to the audience and introduce the person you were sitting next to.

WOW ok, so this was going to be a full-on three days! Now anybody who knows me well knows that I do not go outside of my comfort zone often, if at all. And public speaking, guess what - that was one of my fears.

But I managed to get up on stage and deliver my introduction, without looking completely silly.

Later that afternoon/evening, we needed to deliver a 60-second pitch about what we were hoping to achieve. We were split up into groups; the first group was going to stay and go through their pitches first while the second group went and got dinner, etc. I was in the second group, so we did our pitches later.

Suffice to say my 60-second pitch was more like a 15 second, ahhhh I forgot speech. I'm probably too hard on myself, but that's what it seemed like to me.

Sam came up on stage to critique me and was very positive about what I had to say, which helped immensely.

Fast forward to day two, and we were split up into three groups for the majority of the conference. I was in the black group, and I met the most amazing and sincere people and made some great friendships.

My schizoaffective disorder kicked into overdrive on day two, and with it, my depressive mind started on the whole you're not good enough, you can't do this, go back up to your room and hide. Thankfully, I spoke to Kate Cawthorn (Sam's Wife), and she was so lovely and managed to help me calm down and realise that I would survive.

I got up to deliver my 6-minute presentation and got as far as 2 minutes and 30 seconds. The mentors in the room had me stay up on stage for a bit longer and asked me to relate any story I could think of. They wanted me to get used to being up on stage.

I then delivered the humorous story about Snowy and the computers all going off their heads - you know the one, you read about that in the book earlier :)

We then broke up into smaller groups (five people) and listened to and provided advice to each other about what we could do to make our presentations even better for the final performance on day three (which is professionally recorded).

On day three, I felt so much better in myself and about the message I had that I wanted to get out there about mental health and everyone being so blasé about it most of the time.

I got up on the stage, and I owned it. I'm not one to toot my own horn, but I was thrilled with how it went, and everyone clapped and cheered loudly. It indeed was one of the most life-changing boot camps I attended, and I cannot thank Sam and the team enough for all of the opportunities provided to us, students.

I also try my best to attend Speakers Tribe meetings that are held monthly, as it's a great way of being in the proximity of other like-minded individuals. It also gives us a chance to brush up on our presentation skills by presenting our 60-second pitch to the audience. I'm part of the Victorian tribe, and if you have any interest in professional speaking, I can highly recommend becoming part of the tribe.

So, I've started on my path of helping others by speaking on stage at speaking events, writing this book and setting up my website.

I also want to take other people who are suffering from mental illness on challenges like the Larapinta Trail in Northern Territory or even the Inca Trail in Peru. Since I found my challenge to be indispensable, I feel it would help others as well.

From a personal point of view, the last few years have been very challenging for me.

My mental health has been in a precarious position at times. I've often found days where it was all too much, and I just wanted to crawl into bed and not get out again. My schizoaffective disorder has been in full swing during periods of high stress/anxiety. I have tried a few different medications during the last couple of years, but I have settled back down into my original combination of drugs - Effexor XR and Olanzapine. However, we have added one extra medication, called Mirtazapine. This three-way combination of drugs is keeping me reasonably straight and level and the ability to function daily.

"I'm competitive, and I love to create challenges for myself. Maybe that's not always a good thing.
It can make life complicated."
– Donald Trump

Summary

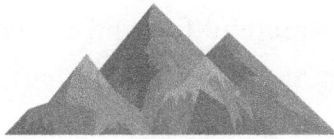

Phew - now that you have read part one, what are your thoughts about it? It sure was a crazy ride, but I don't think I would change it for anything. It's helped shape me into the person I am today, and overall I'm pretty happy with who I am. Sure there are some things I could go back and change, but who knows what ripple effect those changes would cause. That and possibly because time travel hasn't been invented yet, but hey why sweat the small stuff.

There was some definite heavy talk around my suicide attempts, so I'm hoping you're ok right now and it hasn't triggered you. If you found this section of my book particularly difficult and you're not in the best headspace right now, I encourage you – no I implore you - to seek out assistance. There are numerous phone hotlines you can call to discuss things. Make an appointment with your Psychologist or Psychiatrist. If you would like to reach out to me you are more than welcome to do so; the best email is info@craigmarchant.com – just keep in mind I might not be able to get back to you straight away, but I will always answer when I can.

I look back at my life now, with the perspective of all my years since and feel grateful. My life could have certainly been a heck of a lot worse, but of course, when you're in the thick of battle, you rarely have time to indulge in self-reflection.

One thing I am very grateful for, and always will be, has been the love and support of my family. At times, my family was the only thing keeping me going. In the beginning, it was just my family unit, mum, dad, sister, brother and grandparents. As I progressed and started having relationships and kids as part of, these are what keep me going at the end of the day.

I hope that my story will inspire you to reach for the stars as well and aim high. It doesn't matter if you don't achieve everything you plan straight away; don't give up on yourself and above all else be kind to yourself. There are enough people in this world who will try and knock you down, don't be one of them. You can be your own worst enemy, I know I certainly was, and even on occasion I still am.

PART 2

Putting it all into Practice

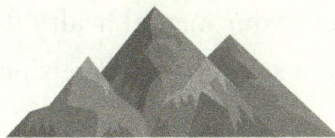

In this upcoming part of my book, we will examine what I believe to be the critical steps to help improve your mental health. Some of them are probably obvious, but others will not be so obvious. Mental health is such a complex subject, and I'm a firm believer that no one person has all the answers. Here, I do my best to guide you on what I feel has been vital to my success.

Just for the record, I have included sections on mental health supports like psychologists and psychiatrists and medications. Not everyone thinks that these are vital to successfully navigating your way out of the black pit of despair. You may agree, or disagree, of course. But what you should take away from this is that mental health illnesses seem to present when undergoing periods of extreme stress and anxiety. Try and simplify your life as best as you can and research and try as many different methods you can to help relieve your mental health illnesses. Remember there is no right way, just your way of getting out from under it.

CHAPTER 1

A Glimmer of Hope

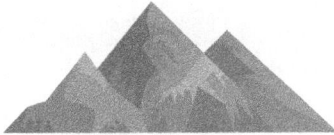

"The Journey of a Thousand Miles Begins
with One Step."
– Lao Tzu

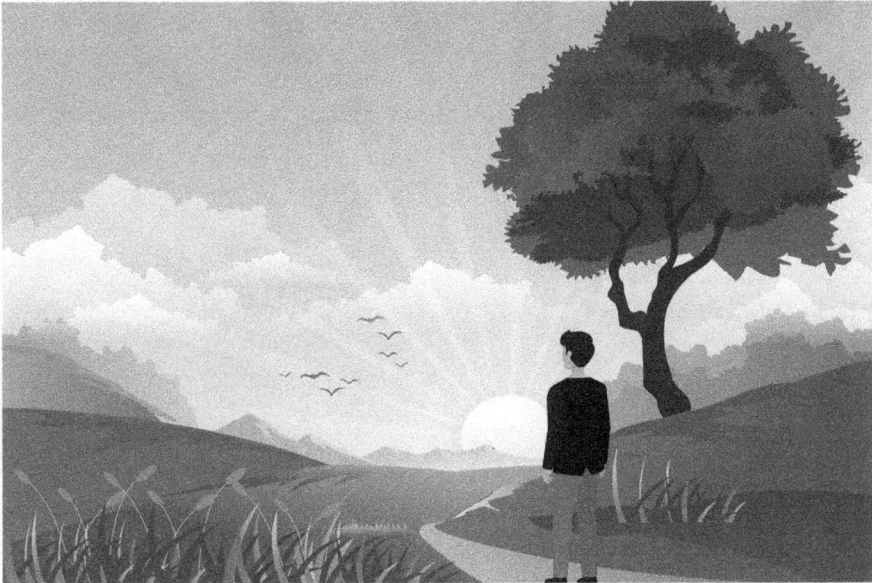

COMMON THOUGHTS

I don't need to see a doctor; I'm just in a bad place at the moment!

While it's true that you could be in a bad place right at the moment, let me ask you a few questions. Has it lasted longer than a few days? Have you noticed any other changes such as sleep disturbances, or feeling useless? It might be more than you think. Of course, the only person who is qualified to tell you if you have depression is your doctor, so it might pay to make an appointment to get assessed.

Real men don't talk about their emotions and feelings!

Real men realise when they need help. There is simply nothing unblokey about getting help.

I'm not a psycho!

Nobody said you were. Just because you are having mental health problems does not make you the next Jeffrey Dahmer or Charles Manson. Plenty of famous people have mental illness conditions, and it hasn't stopped them from living a full life.

Insights

Just as the quote says, making the first step is often the hardest. Your first step should be to reach out to your GP/Physician and make an appointment to see them.

For your first appointment, consider taking a support person along with you. The support person can be anybody you trust - they will be there to support you and also to act as a second pair of ears as there can be a lot of information to take in.

It also helps to write down a list of all your symptoms for the doctor and a list of questions you would like to ask.

Your doctor may decide to prescribe you antidepressants and may also give you a referral to make an appointment with a psychologist or psychiatrist depending on your requirements.

Your GP will also more than likely get you to fill out a quick questionnaire about how you are feeling and will assign a score. It's essential to keep in mind that there are no right or wrong answers or correct score to get - just truthfully answer the questions as best you can. Remember, if you purposefully decide to fill out the questionnaire incorrectly, it will be much harder for your GP to get a complete picture of what is going on.

Ongoing Support

After your initial visit with your GP, you may be seeing them a lot in the next few months. This is because they will want to check in on you and make sure you are ok. It will also be to see how the medication they have prescribed for you (if they did prescribe medication) is doing as well. Keep in mind that it can take several weeks for the medicine to kick in, so don't expect an immediate change in your mood/behaviour.

I have an excellent relationship with my GP at our local practice, so I know I can trust him when it comes to recommendations about my health. Think about it as entering into a partnership; you both work together to create solutions that are tailor-made for you. That could include things like medication, psychologists, exercise and even diet.

Your GP will probably be the one supplying you with your prescriptions and doing a lot of the leg work. If you live in Australia, they will likely complete a Mental Health Plan for you, which you supply to your psychologist and you get up to ten subsidised visits in a calendar year. I am fortunate that my psychologist bulk bills for my appointments, so it doesn't cost me anything upfront. Not all psychologists do this, so it pays to check with your psychologist first when making an appointment, so you are not surprised with a bill at the end of the session.

If you are suffering badly from depression, then you might be eligible for the NDIS - the National Disability Insurance Scheme.

These plans are for a set amount of funding in the review period, usually a year, and can help with things like getting more support for your illness, cleaners, social workers, etc.

While you can complete the application process on your own, many agencies can help you with your application and guide you in the right direction. This might be just what you need if you are suffering from depression anyway as even the simplest things can seem quite daunting and completing the NDIS application form is not simple.

One topic that I would like to discuss further is what to do if your doctor suggests hospitalisation. Even though the first thoughts might be no way in hell is that happening, don't discard the idea altogether.

I have been in a few psychiatric wards before myself and sometimes just like medication - it's the best thing at the time. I remember one time when I was admitted to a psychiatric ward, the doctors were in the middle of changing my medication, and I had some unintended side effects that triggered off my schizoaffective disorder. On this occasion, I couldn't even determine what was real or not, so the hospital was the best place for me for a week or so. I guess what I am trying to say is - don't automatically become defensive and offended should the doctor mention that a hospital stay might be appropriate.

I have personally found that depression seems to come from one of three areas:

- Chemical Imbalance - Your body just isn't making the right chemicals needed.
- Emotional Imbalance - Your lived experiences and responses have helped lead to your depression.
- A combination of both.

For me, my depression seems to be a combination of both chemical and emotional imbalance. Keep in mind that if you are prescribed medications to take - they will hopefully help you but don't be under any illusion that they are a magical cure.

It will help to even out your moods and lighten your depression, but you are still going to need to do some serious therapeutic work with your psychologist/counsellor to get any real benefit from them.

Changing GPs

If you find you don't get along with your GP, don't be afraid to look around for another. You need to be able to trust them to get effective treatment.

I've had a mixed bag when it comes to doctors. Some have been good, and others have had a terrible bedside manner. This isn't to say they aren't good doctors, just not the right ones for me.

Let's say that you have had the same doctor for many years, but at this consultation, you found them to be lacking empathy or compassion. Having a mental illness can make things seem much worse than what they are. My recommendation would be to give them one final shot before moving. Maybe they were just having a bad day, or you were having a bad day or both. It does happen - remember your doctor is a human as well and therefore capable of the same sorts of issues as everybody else.

If you are going to change your GP, then you probably need to organise to get a copy of any relevant reports/results so you can give them to your new doctor. You might be lucky and see a different doctor at the same clinic as your old doctor, in which case they should be able to access all of your medical records without having to get copies faxed/emailed.

Your new GP should be able to get you to sign an authority to release which can be faxed over to the old doctor's clinic and then have the required information released.

Just recently, Australia has brought out the MyHealthRecord system, which is an electronic system for storing medical information about you and your conditions, etc. Some practices have this information being continuously uploaded and others not so much. You can ask your GP if it's possible to upload your history to the system.

You are also able to see what details are held on file with the MyHealthRecord system, by logging in via the myGov website and clicking on the MyHealthRecord section.

"I Like the Night. Without the Dark,
We'd Never See the Stars."
– Stephanie Meyer

Summary

We discussed the first steps to getting help which begins with your GP/Doctor. You should also write down your symptoms and take a support person with you if you can. We talked about prescribed medications and covered some basic do and don'ts. We discussed ongoing support and how depression can come from either an emotional imbalance, a chemical imbalance or both in many cases. We discussed if you should need to change your GP/Doctor due to them not being the right fit for you and finally about the MyHealthRecord system here in Australia.

Action Plan

- Book an appointment with your GP
- See if a support person can accompany you to your appointment
- Make a list of your symptoms and issues to tell your GP
- Ask your GP any questions you have.

CHAPTER 2

Opening Your Pillbox

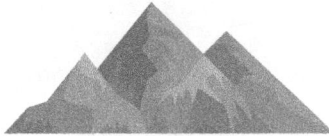

"Always Laugh When You Can -
It Is Cheap Medicine."
– Lord Byron

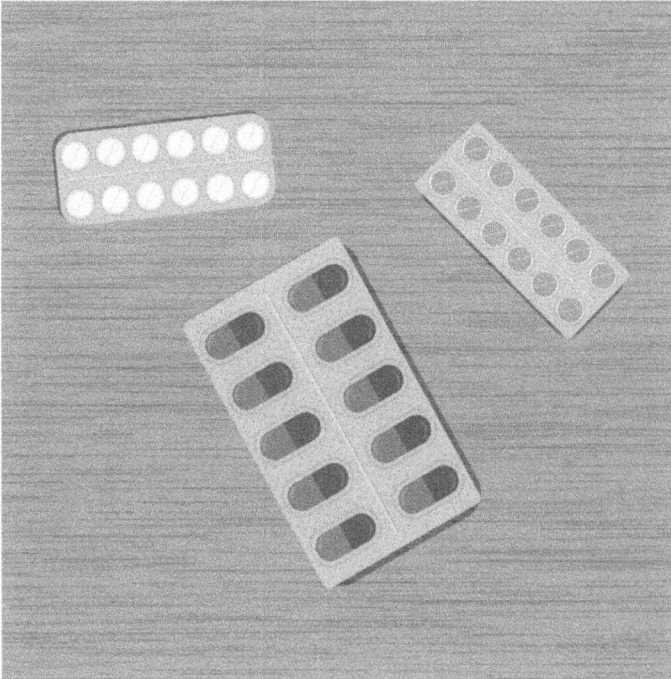

COMMON THOUGHTS

I'm not taking medication, why should I just to be normal!

This is an objection I hear all too often, and if I'm honest, I used to think the same way as well. Why the hell should I have to take medications just to make me a normal human being? Yep, it's true that it kind of sucks however you need to look at it from a different point of view. If you had diabetes and had to go on medication, you would more than likely do it without a second thought. Depression/Anxiety is just like diabetes in that it's an illness. Both are treatable and help you live a full and active life.

I don't want to be on medication for the rest of my life!

This is another objection that I hear way too often, and yes, I have to put my hand up again and say this was another little gem I used to tell myself all the time. Once again, I'm going to use diabetes as a comparison. While it's true that a lot of people who have diabetes will have to stay on medications for the rest of their lives, some get a second chance and can stop it. Depression medication is similar in that you probably won't need to be on it forever. For me, I will more than likely have to take it for the rest of my life, but I'm more the exception, not the rule.

I've read about the side effects of taking medications, and I'm worried about them!

Yes, some of the medicines can have side effects. Sometimes those side effects will be only small things and other times bigger things. If a specific medication is causing too many side effects, then speak with your doctor about changing your medications. There is no reason you have to stay on a particular medicine if it's causing more harm than good. Using me as an example, I do have some side effects that give me trouble. One is sleep – I'm very tired of the morning, and it takes about an hour or two for me to wake up fully. However, I accept that side effect because taking medicine means I can function normally for the rest of the day. A small price to pay I feel.

Insights

As you would have read in the previous chapters, I take several medications that help me maintain my mental health. I'm not ashamed to admit this as without the medication, I have a lot of problems and struggle to function correctly.

I'm currently taking 10mg of Olanzapine (Zyprexa) to help control the schizophrenic symptoms, and I take a combination of 300mg of Venlafaxine (Effexor XR) and 15mg of Mirtazapine to combat the depression symptoms. That combination of antidepressants is referred to as "Californian Rocket Fuel".

If you're anything like I was, you may even have an issue with being on medication. My thought was that I hate needing something to make me function properly. But then I started looking at it from the point of view that mental illness is like any other illness and if that's what you need to do, so be it.

It should be noted that finding the right medication is often a case of trial and error. You might hit on the right one straight away, or it might take a couple of times before you find the right one. Always listen to and seek the advice of your doctors.

When your doctor first puts you on medication, it can take several weeks for antidepressants to kick in and start working. During this time, you are more susceptible to suicidal thoughts and self-harm behaviours. But I would say to you, hang in there - it does get better I promise.

If you're being prescribed a new medication to take, my advice is to start it on a Friday night. Don't plan to do much over the weekend, and if you have to drive, be careful. Some of the medications have an unfortunate side effect of making you drowsy and just starting on them; this goes doubly true. I found by the time Monday morning rolled around things were much better.

SSRI and SNRI medications are the newer type that generally have fewer side effects to the old school TCA's. But you shouldn't panic if you are put on a TCA. Your doctor is the best person to decide as to what you need to use.

So, what exactly are some of these medications that you could potentially be put on? I've created a list of them and added them to my website. You can access by going to https://www.craigmarchant.com/resources

Please note that this is not a complete list of medications used to treat depression. Also, this doesn't list any of the schizophrenia medications.

Side Effects

All medications have side effects which can range from mild to severe. I have never experienced anything more than mild side effects from any of the medicines I have taken. But just because it's never happened to me, that doesn't mean it won't happen for you.

I take my medications in the evening, as they have a sedative effect on me. I still find it very difficult to wake up in the morning and often I'm somewhat hazy for the first hour or two even with taking it early in the evening.

It's all a case of trial and error until you find the right method for you.

Side effects can be unpleasant, and I've been told the first seven to ten days are the worst. Just hang in there, after that period everything should start to calm down for you. At least that's what I have found in my personal experience.

Long Term Usage and Withdrawal Symptoms

I would, however, caution you against a particular type of activity while on the medications. Do not under any circumstances, stop taking your medications without a thorough discussion with your GP/Doctor. It can cause some very unpleasant side effects while you are coming off them. I speak from experience; I have come off them many times while I still objected to the thought of being on medications. Just trust me on this one, don't do it.

I recall a conversation I had with one of my psychiatrists at the time, and we were discussing how I wasn't happy that I needed to have this medication to help me be "normal". I mentioned to him that it seemed to be that I come off them and I'm ok for a while and then have to go back on them for one reason or another.

He said to me, "Craig; you are what I call a lifer - you will need to be on medications for the rest of your life because of how long you have had depression". I wasn't exactly thrilled with the particular prospect of that, but it is what it is.

Something else to think about is not to mix certain types of medications. For example, some medications cannot be taken with others because there is a chance for a condition called Serotonin Syndrome to develop. This is a dangerous condition which can cause high body temperature, agitation, increased reflexes, tremors, sweating and a whole bunch of other symptoms that are not good.

As long as you follow the advice of your doctor, there should be no issues. Should you develop any of the symptoms above, let your doctor know or get yourself to your local hospital for evaluation.

Final Thoughts

If you want to know more about any medications you are taking, there are a few options. You can ask your doctor, your pharmacist, and finally, you can ask good old Google. Just be a little wary about taking anything verbatim from the internet. While there are some excellent sites out there, there are some dodgy ones as well.

If you have trouble remembering to take your medication, I can recommend a few different methods to help you remember.

Pillboxes are a great idea, as they have the day written on them and will help you to know if you have already taken them. It also helps with remembering to take them. Another great idea is to get your local pharmacy to Webster pack your medications, especially if you have to take a lot of different medicines.

You can also ask a support person (ideally someone you live with) to remind you to take your medications.

Finally, there are apps you can get on your phone to remind you to take your medications. Some of these apps can also double to remind you when your scripts are getting low and you need to visit the doctor to get repeats. I use the "Chemist Warehouse" app, because that's the closest pharmacy to home and they keep all my scripts on file, so I know exactly when I'm getting low and need refills or need to get repeat scripts. It seems a lot of the pharmacies have their own apps now, so check out your phone's app store.

"Let Food Be Thy Medicine and
Medicine Be Thy Food."
– Hippocrates

Summary

We discussed that finding the right medication for your mental illness can be a case of trial and error sometimes and that all medicines have side effects, it just depends on what you will have. We talked about long term usage and withdrawal symptoms if you do need to come off your medication. We briefly spoke about Serotonin Syndrome and what to do if you develop any of the symptoms mentioned, and we finished up with some helpful tips on taking your medications.

Action Plan

- Finding the right medication for you
- Ask your GP/Doctor about any potential side effects of your medication
- Ask your Doctor/Pharmacist for an info sheet for your medication
- Check my website for further information
- Use Google for more info but remember Google doesn't always know everything and you can't always believe everything that Google says. Remember, well-meaning people can post incorrect information.

CHAPTER 3

Expanding Your Medical Team

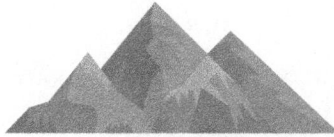

"Knowing yourself is the beginning of all wisdom."
– Aristotle

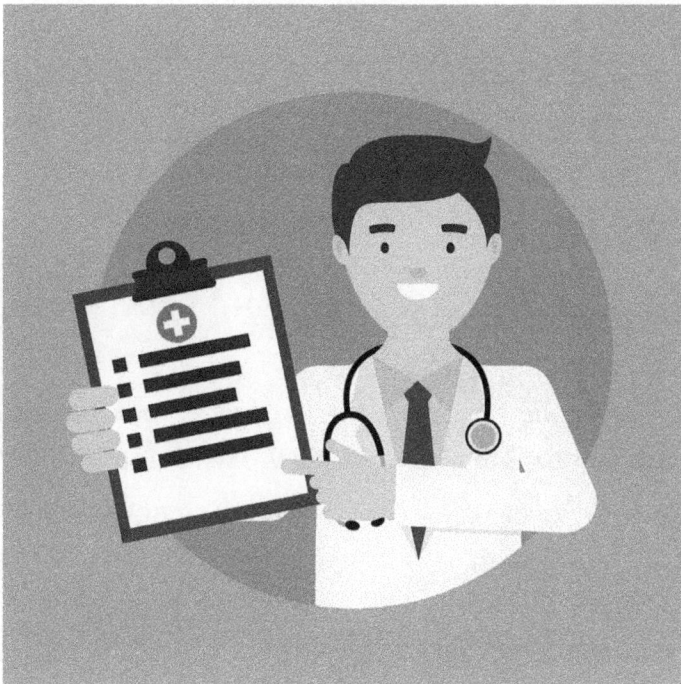

COMMON THOUGHTS

I am not going to see a psychologist! I don't like discussing my problems.

To get better, you are going to need to be able to discuss your problems with your therapist. They can't even begin to imagine how stressful certain life events have been for you without you guiding them in the right direction. Think of it as a mutually beneficial arrangement. They find out what issues you have and then can give you different ways of handling the situation.

Only loonies see shrinks!

You might be surprised at how many people see therapists and how beneficial they find this. I wholeheartedly believe that everyone could benefit from having somebody to talk to that can offer you a different perspective/outside view.

What will everyone think of me?

Let's be honest here - nobody is going to find out you are visiting a therapist unless you tell them. And it's kind of a private thing, and it's up to you who and when you tell anybody about it. I would encourage you to speak to your partner/spouse about it so you can talk freely about those sessions. I often find speaking with my wife after the event helps to cement the session fully in my mind.

Insights

I have had a few psychologists and psychiatrists in my life. They are both equally as important if you ask me, although they don't always get the appreciation they deserve.

There is a stigma associated with seeing these sort of doctors as if it's some sort of shameful activity. There is no shame in recognising that you have an illness and need assistance. Your brain is just like your body, a sophisticated machine that may need tuning sometimes.

Ask your GP/Doctor for recommendations about a reputable psychologist or psychiatrist. They are not all equal; some have a terrible bedside manner and don't encourage any meaningful conversation and let's face it - if you want to get better, you're going to need to look into the deepest parts of your soul and spill the beans. You're not likely to do that if you cannot stand your team.

Your doctor may have referred you to a psychologist or psychiatrist. I'm here to tell you if you get referred to one or both, then definitely don't delay. While I'm not sure how it fares in the rest of the world, here in Australia, there can be a significant delay in getting into either of them.

What's the Difference Between Psychologist and Psychiatrist?

They each perform a different type of service, however, psychologists generally do not prescribe medications; however, they can, of course, make recommendations to your GP or psychiatrist.

Just because you're not suffering from any schizophrenia symptoms, it doesn't mean you won't be referred to a psychiatrist sometimes. Since they specialise in medications for mental illness as well as schizophrenia and other psychiatric disorders, it makes them the perfect person to review and suggest changes to your medication should it be needed.

How Often Will I See Them?

I have regular sessions with my psychologist, usually about one each month. The psychiatrist I see far less often at the moment - usually once a year to review medications and to see how I am going.

You may see your psychologist more frequently in the beginning while they do the initial groundwork. There is nothing wrong if they want to see you more often; be guided by them.

It took a while to find a psychologist that I work well with. You may get lucky and on the first go and find somebody who you click with, or you might need to try your luck with a few different ones before finding your ultimate one.

While we are discussing how often you will see your psychologist or psychiatrist, let's talk about the rise of Telehealth services which kicked into gear during the great COVID-19 pandemic in 2020.

Telehealth Services

As you would be aware, the COVID-19 pandemic kicked off in early 2020, and by mid-March, most of Australia was being advised to self-isolate for their safety. If you were landing back in the country, you were transferred to hotels to serve a 14-day mandatory lockdown. A whole raft of restrictions were introduced to slow the spread of the virus.

As you can probably imagine, mental health services along with all other types of services were affected and there needed to be a new way of being able to continue to see your psychologist/psychiatrist or indeed any doctor during this time.

Queue the rise of Telehealth services, where you would use your computer or mobile phone and an active internet connection to connect virtually with your health practitioner. The jury is still out on how effective this will be and how long it will last. My guess is that Telehealth is here to stay and won't be going anywhere in a hurry. It is especially useful for those living in more rural areas where accessing healthcare services is especially tricky.

One area that will need to be streamlined will be prescriptions for medications. It simply will not be realistic to wait for a doctor's prescription to be sent to you physically via the mail – a system where it can be sent electronically to your local pharmacy will be needed. I believe this can be done already via faxing, but it's a tedious process for all involved, and you still need to give the real prescription to the pharmacy when it arrives.

What Do You Talk About?

I discuss anything and everything that pops up, along with a quick catch up with what we spoke about previously in our sessions. I recall one particular conversation I had with my psychiatrist at the time who was asking me exactly how I felt and what was going on. At this point, I was feeling very down and had thoughts about suicide. I expressed those thoughts to him, and he decided that I needed to go into a psychiatric ward in a hospital for a while. I didn't want to go, however, was advised that because of my disclosure I needed to go, and he wasn't going to take no for an answer.

For the record, I was in the hospital for about a week, and then I got out of there. It was a real eye-opener for me - I could see people who had it far worse than I did in there. At least I can tell when I see and hear things that aren't there, unlike those poor people who cannot tell.

But you shouldn't take this to mean that you shouldn't say how you are feeling, quite the opposite. If you are feeling so God-awful, then tell them. You want to be safe, and if you can't guarantee that safety, then the hospital is the best place for you.

What Is Your Schizoaffective Disorder Like?

I don't often speak about what I see and hear with my schizoaffective disorder; however, I feel it might be useful for others to know.

When I hear voices, they are telling me that I'm no good, and I should just kill myself and do everyone a favour. Or variants of that recurring theme. They are always negative but have never told me to hurt anybody but myself.

What I see is far more interesting. I see walls coated in blood, floating heads and long since passed relatives. I like to describe it as a horror movie playing out from my eyes.

One of the computer games that I played "Quest for Glory 4" has a character called Domovoi. During one of my episodes, which seem to come on when I have a reasonably high fever mainly, I was trying to convince my daughter Jasmine that Domovoi was sitting on the car's dashboard and that she had to look after it for me.

I always find it amazing how resilient children can be. My wife Kendyl was out at a baby shower, and I was home alone with Chelsea, Jasmine and Zachery. The kids had to call my mum, who then called Kendyl to come back. It would have been a scary thing for the kids to witness, but they handled it quite well. I spoke to them about it afterwards so they could understand what was going on.

Stigma and Controversy

There is a misconception in the community and society that those of us who have psychotic illnesses such as schizoaffective disorder and schizophrenia are violent and dangerous and should be avoided at all costs. The media, unfortunately, does little to help dispel that notion at times with careless reporting. I do not think it is intentional on their part, just perhaps a limited understanding of the true nature of our illness.

Some people who do have these illnesses do get violent and aggressive on occasion, but the vast majority of us are actually very kind and gentle and would never hurt anybody. These media reports often leave us feeling alone and pretty much not understood at all.

I can understand that it can be somewhat disconcerting for somebody who does not have these illnesses to perhaps witness somebody talking to themselves or being incoherent. What can you say to somebody who is having a conversation with themselves? Well, I would like to put forth a novel idea – a simple "Hello" or "Hi, how are you?". Something so simple might just have the most profound effect on the person you are saying it to. They may or may not return the conversation, but I can assure you – deep down the person knows and suddenly feels a little less alone in the world.

When somebody says "mental illness" they often think automatically of depression, forgetting that there are a wide range of mental illnesses out there that are not depression. It is great that we as a society have become more accepting of people suffering from depression and suicide, and now there are a number of support services out there to help deal with that. But what we now need to work on is accepting just as much those who have the "other" mental health illnesses, and provide the necessary support for them.

"In my opinion, our health care system has failed when a doctor fails to treat an illness that Is treatable."
– Kevin Alan Lee

Summary

We discussed the stigma associated with mental illness and getting recommendations for reputable psychologists/psychiatrists. We discussed the differences between the two specialists and how often you will see them. We talked about the rise of Telehealth services during the COVID-19 pandemic and how they are probably here to stay. We discussed what you talk about when you see your psychologist/psychiatrist, which for the record is anything and everything. And finally, we wrapped up with me describing my schizoaffective disorder and the stigma and controversies created by the media sometimes.

Action Plan

- Finding the right medication for you
- Ask your GP/Doctor about any potential side effects of your medication
- Ask your Doctor/Pharmacist for an info sheet for your medication
- Check my website for further information.

CHAPTER 4

Somewhere in the Great Outdoors

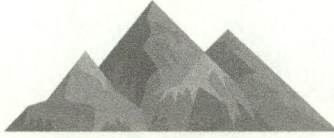

"Live in the sunshine, swim in the sea,
drink the wild air."

– Ralph Waldo Emerson

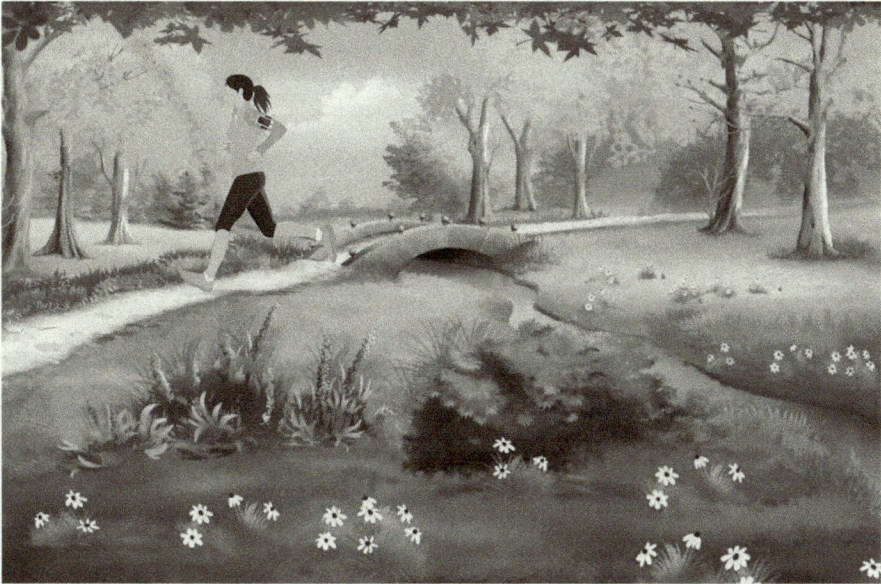

COMMON THOUGHTS

I'm just too heavy to start exercising; I need to lose some weight first!

> *Yes, I've also said the same thing before. But you know what, even just a gentle walk can make a world of difference. You don't need to go all out to make a difference.*

I've got an injury which prevents me from participating in exercise.

> *This was a common excuse I used myself when trying to avoid exercise. If you have a knee or ankle injury, sure walking or jogging might just be way too much for your joints, but you can try something else like going for a swim at the local pool as an example.*

I'm not overweight/unhealthy, so why do I even need to exercise?

> *While you may not be overweight or think yourself unhealthy, exercising releases endorphins which give you a natural high. It will also give you a sense of accomplishment that you achieved something that day if nothing else.*

Insights

If you are Australian, you might remember Ernie Dingo from The Great Outdoors on your television with his signature catchphrase - "And I'll see you somewhere in the great outdoors". I used to love watching it, so many different places they would explore and discover.

Our planet is truly a wonder to behold, and you should try and explore it as much as possible. It doesn't matter where you live in the world; almost every country has some spectacular experiences just waiting for you.

The next time I'm in the United States of America I'm aiming to do a trek of the Grand Canyon on some of their majestic trails. It is high on my list of things to do. Also high on my list is to hike up Mt Kilimanjaro in Africa and The Great Wall of China.

As you would have read earlier in my book, back in 2016, I trekked the Inca Trail in Peru for the Leukaemia Foundation. I did a lot of preparation for the trail; I did the 1000 steps a few times, which is the Kokoda Track Memorial Walk in the Dandenong Ranges National Park in Victoria - beautiful views but a real workout.

I also did a lot of walking beforehand, and there are a few walking trails near our place. A lap around our estate lasts about 30 minutes and is around 2km. The walking trails are approximately one to two hours, depending on the track taken.

And with all of this, I still found the Inca Trail to be super challenging. The combination of being outdoors, getting good exposure to sunlight and fresh air did absolute wonders for my mental health.

Benefits of Getting Outside

Did you know that exercise, while making you fitter, will also help you feel better? Your psychologist or counsellor will probably tell you this, but if not, I will.

By getting outside, you will start to feel better - exercise releases endorphins which makes you happier and helps contribute to you losing weight.

Part of your recovery should include some form of exercise. It doesn't have to be anything complicated or over the top - 15 to 30 minutes of light exercise a couple of times a week will do wonders for your mental health.

You also get the bonus of getting some sunlight exposure which is responsible for your Vitamin D levels. Seasonal Affective Disorder is a particular type of depression that occurs in the Autumn and Winter months of the year. The current thought pattern as to why this happens is because there is less light in those seasons generally. So, getting outside and having some sunlight exposure will do wonders for you and your mental health.

Outdoor Activities

- Go for a walk along the beach. You also get the bonus of being able to turn around and see just how far you have travelled.
- Go for a walk around your estate. You can even listen to some music while you are walking. Trust me; it helps make the distance seem shorter.
- Go outside and play with your kids.
- Go for a bushwalk or nature walk. It's free to walk, and you get to experience different places such as national and local parks.
- Ride a bike. This helps reduce pressure on your joints.
- Swimming is another excellent way to get in some exercise. Swimming is also a suitable exercise method when you can't place a lot of weight on your joints.
- You can get some incidental walking in merely by going to a wildlife preserve or zoo. All the walking around will be great exercise. I'm also kind of partial to seeing the Penguins at Phillip Island in Victoria, Australia. Make sure you check it out once in your life.
- I will also be taking small groups of participants on adventure challenges, such as the Larapinta Trail in the NT, The Inca Trail in Peru, South America and even the Great Wall of China. These are fantastic ways to get in exercise, but also do something amazing for your mental health and wellbeing.

With the medications I'm on, the first few hours of the day are my most challenging. If I'm just sitting around doing nothing, then I feel awful along with being tired and groggy. However, if I'm doing some physical activities like mowing the lawn or going for a walk, I seem to fare much better.

Where to Start

Have you decided to get some exercise in? Fantastic! But where do you start? Well, there are a few essential/optional items which might make things a bit easier for you.

Firstly, make sure you have a water bottle on hand when you are exercising. When you exercise, you sweat, and that means you need to re-hydrate often. Water is an excellent way of doing just that, and bonus it has zero calories! If you are going to be exercising for an extended period, it might pay to have a bottle of Powerade or Gatorade on hand as well, since these drinks also replenish essential minerals and vitamins.

You might find a Fitbit or Smartwatch to be an excellent investment as well. These can record your heart rate, how far you have walked, calories burned and a whole host of other cool features. While it's not essential to have this, it's a handy addition to your arsenal if you can afford it.

If you haven't done much exercise in a fair while, you don't want to rush straight into a gruelling workout. It's recommended that you check in with your GP first to make sure you are in decent shape before starting any exercise regime.

I would advise you to do a five or ten-minute session for a couple of days until your body starts getting used to it. Then you can increase the frequency and duration to suit your unique requirements.

If you want to incorporate more walking into your daily life, things like getting off the train or bus one stop before yours will allow you to get some walking in. You could also park your car further away at the shops to get in some extra exercise.

If you are a private person and prefer not to exercise in public, I would recommend you get yourself a treadmill if you can afford one, or even walking around your backyard will help.

You can also try to convince one of your mates/friends to join you in your quest for better health and that way you have somebody you can talk with while you are exercising.

The American Heart Association recommends getting approximately 150 minutes per week of moderate-intensity aerobic activity or 75 minutes of high-intensity aerobic exercise. They even recommend switching it up so that you get a mix of the two.

"Adopt the Pace of Nature:
Her Secret Is Patience."
– Ralph Waldo Emerson

Summary

We talked about the importance of getting some exercise into your schedule. We discussed how I had to do a lot of training for the Inca Trail and how, even with that training, I still found it to be super challenging. We discussed the benefits of exercise and how it helps with Seasonal Affective Disorder. We talked about the different activities you can do to get some exercise. And finally, we talked about how you can get started.

Action Plan

- Based on your own unique goals and situation, work out which of the activities listed above or that you can think of for yourself that will suit you.
- Start small, don't go all out straight away - you need time to build up to a lot of exercise.
- Consider purchasing or using a Fitbit or Smartwatch to help record your vitals and distance/calories while you are exercising.
- Remember you can get in extra exercise by parking further away.
- Above all else, enjoy yourself. Why be miserable if you don't have to?

CHAPTER 5

You Are What You Eat

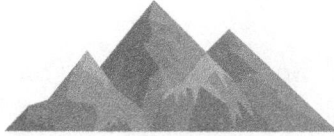

"All you need is love. But a little chocolate now and then doesn't hurt."

– Charles M. Schulz

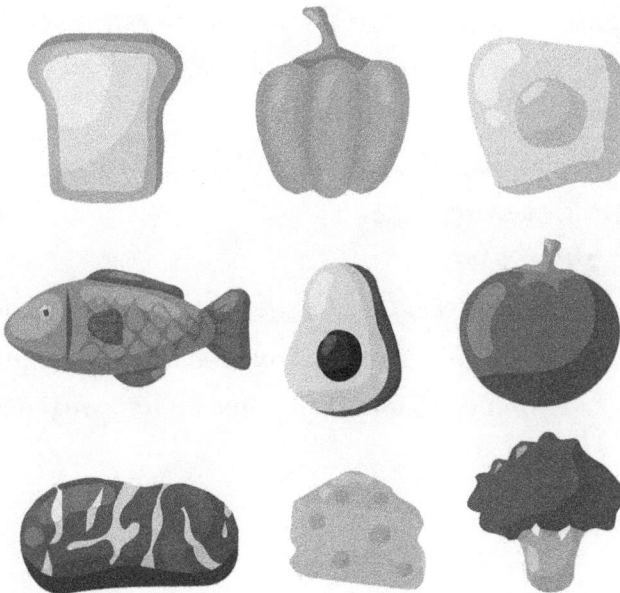

COMMON THOUGHTS

I'm currently at my ideal weight, why should I be worried about diet?

Even though you might be at your ideal weight, consuming foods and drinks that are not good for you may contribute to your overall mood. You want all the help you can get when it comes to your mental health.

I'm currently overweight, having put on many kilos since starting treatment. What should I do?

Do NOT stop taking your medication abruptly. You need to talk it out with your GP and work out a new battle plan if you're struggling with the side effects.

In your personal view, would you recommend weight loss surgery?

Just because it hasn't been a silver bullet for me, it doesn't mean that it won't work for you. You need to weigh up all the pro's and con's and then make an informed decision for yourself.

Insights

Numerous studies have concluded that the food you eat and drinks you consume can directly affect the brain both positively and negatively. Nutritional psychiatry is an emerging field that investigates the role of food and drinks in mental health. The foods and drinks you consume cause your digestive tract to react, which in turn then affects your brain and ultimately leads to your mood.

If you consume high-quality foods and drinks, then you are giving yourself the best chance of maintaining better mental health. However, when you are depressed, there is a good chance you will make poorer food and beverage choices, which leads to adverse changes in your mood. In other words, it's a vicious cycle.

It's very common to put on weight when you are depressed, mainly because of medication but also because you're more likely to say, stuff it; I'm going to eat junk that I normally might not. And generally, those foods and drinks are going to be loaded with excess sugar and carbohydrates. Antidepressants and antipsychotics are notorious for weight gain. There is no real way to determine precisely what side effects you are going to experience; you just have to roll with the punches.

When you are depressed, it's much harder to lose weight because of the possible poor choices in food and drinks and then the bonus of not feeling motivated to do a single thing about it. Let's cover a few of the things that you can do to maintain a healthy and nutritional diet.

Diet

Foods and drinks that can help improve your mood include:

- Salmon and tuna as they help provide Omega-3 fatty acids which the body cannot generate on its own
- Dark chocolate
- Fermented foods such as kimchi, yogurt, kefir, kombucha and sauerkraut
- Bananas
- Oats such as oatmeal, muesli and granola
- Berries such as blueberries and raspberries
- Nuts and seeds
- Coffee (good news for us coffee lovers)
- Beans and lentils.

If you are time-poor and struggling to come up with healthy meals and snacks, there are numerous companies that double as weight loss solutions as well, including the likes of HelloFresh and Lite n' Easy.

Our family recently tried a HelloFresh box which came with five meals for up to four people (adult servings), so it was perfect for us. It also was a great bonding experience because my eldest daughter Chelsea helped me to prepare and cook the meals, and they were delicious. There wasn't a single meal that wasn't great.

While I enjoy cooking, I do find it rather stressful when trying new recipes for the first time. My anxiety plays up and makes it very challenging. Once I have done a recipe a few times, my anxiety departs, and it's not an issue. I'm not sure if anyone else suffers from the same anxiety when cooking. Surely, I'm not the only one?

If you're not a fan of pre-packaged food and recipes and would prefer to cook your own, I suggest a consultation with a nutritionist/ Dietician. They will be able to tailor an eating plan to your specific requirements.

In Australia, you can see a dietician as part of your mental health plan, so make sure you discuss this with your doctor if it's something you would like to do.

Foods and Drinks to Avoid

Eating foods high in sugars are not good for you - you might feel a bit perkier for a little while, but when you crash - and you will crash - you will feel God-awful. You should also aim to reduce the number of processed foods you consume as they are not suitable for you either.

I don't know about you, but I found it extraordinary that drinking lots of soda/fizzy drinks contributed to my weight gain so much. Example, I'm just looking at a can of Mother Energy Drink. It has a whopping 74.1 grams of sugar in it! A teaspoon generally has 4 grams of sugar in it, so the can of Mother (500ml) has approximately 19 teaspoons of sugar. Holy moly, you have to be kidding me! I don't often drink Mother anymore, but I can see why my weight gain went into overdrive. I used to have a can a day (sometimes two if I'm perfectly honest) so I was consuming so much refined sugar!

Combine that with unsavoury eating habits brought on by being depressed and mood, and it's very easy to see how you can self-sabotage your weight.

It's also a great idea to avoid alcohol while you are on any medication, and probably best to avoid it entirely regardless. While it might make you feel more relaxed, it can react with your medication and make you quite sick. Not to mention a terrible hangover which you don't need on top of everything else.

Emotional Eating and Eating Disorders

I am what is called an emotional eater, where I will eat to alleviate emotional disturbances or even if I'm plain bored. As bad as it sounds, I can sit there in front of the computer and eat an entire bag of corn chips or regular chips in one sitting without giving it any thought whatsoever.

Having a lot of snack/junk foods in your house can present a significant barrier to you being able to maintain or lose weight. Even to this day, I will favour foods that are simple and convenient over foods that are better for me but take slightly longer to prepare. If you are that sort of person, try and reduce the number of junk foods in your house so that there is less temptation for you to conquer.

On the other hand, some people will not feel like eating at all. You need to remember to continue to eat at mealtimes, to avoid developing an eating disorder such as anorexia or bulimia.

Anorexia is a mental illness, just like depression or schizophrenia are, and can have devastating consequences to your physical health and wellbeing. Low body weight and body image issues are hallmarks of this illness. Often the sufferer will have an obsessive fear of gaining weight and will starve their body as a direct result. It is also common for the patient to initiate an increase in exercise levels.

On the other hand, bulimia is another common mental illness where sufferers will binge eat or consume abnormally large amounts of food, and this is then typically followed by self-induced vomiting, fasting and exercising. Generally, this type of illness is more challenging to diagnose since there is every chance the patient is maintaining an average weight or just slightly above/below their ideal body weight.

It's important to know that both of these illnesses constitute a serious issue and should be treated with the utmost attention. These illnesses have a higher rate of death compared with other mental health disorders. One of my daughters recently had a problem with eating, and the treating psychiatrist explained to me that each of the major organs in the body has its own store of energy - think of it as a pantry. When you are not consuming enough calories, your organs are forced to take what they need from those stores. Eventually, those stores will deplete, and then your organs start to suffer as a result. As an example, your heart can get out of rhythm and ultimately lead to heart complications.

Weight Loss Surgery

While weight loss surgery sounds fantastic and easy, nothing could be further from the truth. You still need a lot of willpower and determination to make weight loss surgery successful. A positive mindset is also another qualifying factor.

Firstly, I had the gastric band fitted back in 2014, and I had that for approximately six to eight months. I did manage to lose quite a bit of weight on it, but in the end, it wasn't the right weight loss surgery option for me, so in 2015 I moved to the gastric sleeve. First, I had to have the gastric band removed and had to wait a few months to allow things to settle down before the weight loss doctor would perform the gastric sleeve for me.

At my heaviest, I was approximately 200kgs, which works out at 440 pounds for those using the imperial system. The lowest weight I have achieved is approximately 120kgs, or 264 pounds. So, I managed to lose 80kgs using the gastric sleeve.

One of the reasons the gastric sleeve was so successful for me, well before going back onto my meds, is because when they remove a fair bit of your stomach, they also remove the gastric fundus. The gastric fundus cells are primarily responsible for the production of ghrelin, and ghrelin is known as the "hunger hormone". So obviously, a reduction in the hunger hormone means you are going to eat and store less.

A study on Olanzapine and circulating ghrelin levels found that all participants of the study had increased body fat percentage and serum leptin levels. There was also an increase in both total plasma ghrelin and active ghrelin levels. Six out of the seven patients also reported increased appetites. The study was on a small selection of patients, so while it is interesting, it is in no way 100% indicative[1].

Unfortunately, with having to go back on my Zyprexa (Olanzapine) and the rest of my medication regime, I have put about 50kg's back on at this stage. I'm busy working on getting my mental health back to a good state, and then I'm going to try and continue my weight loss journey and lose this excess weight. My ultimate goal is to get down to about 90kg's. I would be thrilled at that point.

Of course this does raise an interesting question, one which I haven't been able to satisfy myself with either. If the Gastric Fundus is mostly to completely gone due to the sleeve procedure I underwent, then why is the Olanzapine causing weight gain? I did some research and found that small amounts of Ghrelin

---

[1] Murashita M, Kusumi I, Inoue T, et al. Olanzapine increases plasma ghrelin level in patients with schizophrenia. *Psychoneuroendocrinology.* 2005;30(1):106-110. doi:10.1016/j.psyneuen.2004.05.008

https://pubmed.ncbi.nlm.nih.gov/15358448/

are also made by the small intestine, pancreas, and the brain[2]. Maybe the Olanzapine is stimulating one of these other organs into producing higher levels again? It is a theory, but I am not a medical research scientist so I will leave those discoveries to others.

As a fun side note, I lost around 10 kilos while in Peru doing the Inca Trail in 2016. I wasn't able to eat a lot for some reason; it almost seemed like the altitude was shrinking my stomach further and not allowing me to eat much. Either that or the huge amount of exercise I was doing was simply curbing my appetite in a big way. One of the big things that managed to keep me going on the trail was just plain lollies (glucose input)—but I still burned through some serious kg's.

Medications

As mentioned previously, antidepressants and antipsychotics are notorious for weight gain for a lot of people. If I had not had to go back onto my antipsychotics, there is a good chance I would not have put back so much weight on.

The weight gain is a highly undesirable symptom, however when you look at the other option - I would choose to be overweight, but happy and able to function versus being slim but an absolute basket case!

I checked with my GP if it was possible to get a prescription weight loss medication to see if I could shift some of the weight.

---

[2] https://www.yourhormones.info/hormones/ghrelin/

However, he informed me that the weight loss medication would interact negatively with my anti-psychotics medicines, so that is a no go for me.

Should your weight gains become a severe problem for you, then you can always discuss with your GP about changing medications. There is a vast selection of anti-depressants available on the market.

"One Cannot Think Well, Love Well, Sleep Well, If
One Has Not Dined Well."
– Virginia Woolf

Summary

In this chapter, we discussed that when you are depressed, you are more likely to make mediocre food and beverage choices, which can lead to weight gain. We talked about the psychological illnesses of anorexia and bulimia and how they can be life-threatening. We discussed foods and drinks that are good for you and can help with not only your mental health but your gut health as well. There was talk about weight loss surgery and how having a positive mindset and being mentally strong are requirements for a successful surgery. We briefly discussed the role and effects medication can have on your body.

Action Plan

- Assess your current dietary intake and see where you can improve or modify it to make it healthier.
- Be aware that overeating and undereating can be side effects from your medication and that you need to pay particular attention to your weight. If you gain or lose weight, you should let your doctor know.
- Weight loss surgery is an option open to you if you are very overweight and are unable to shift the weight via other means. Do keep in mind, however, that it's not a magic cure and you still need to do some serious work to shift the weight.
- Keep in mind that your medications may cause undesired weight gain or loss. If this becomes concerning, speak to your doctor about changing medications.

CHAPTER 6

Yearning for the Dream World

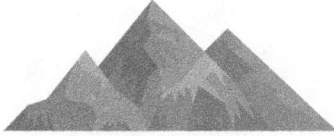

"I love sleep. My life has the tendency to fall apart when I'm awake, you know?"

– Ernest Hemingway

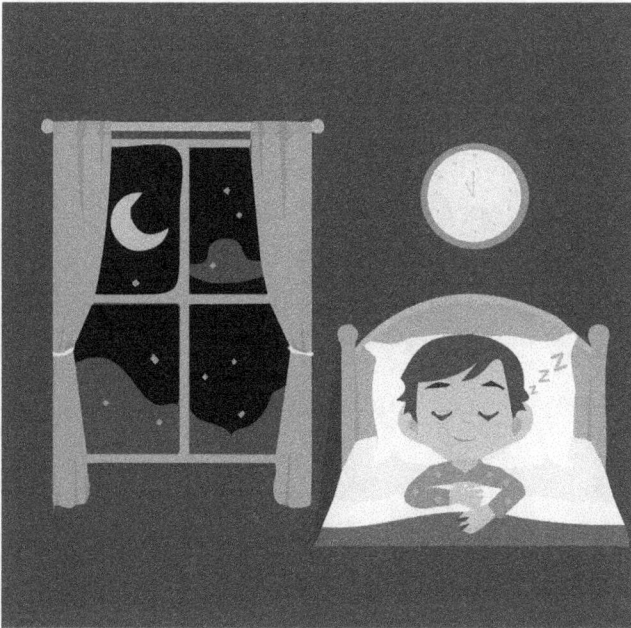

COMMON THOUGHTS

There is nothing wrong with my sleep; I sleep the whole night.

You may be sleeping the entire night, but the quality of your sleep might not be so good. If you have obstructive sleep apnoea, for example, you might be waking up dozens of times each night and not even realise it. If this is the case, you probably feel more tired when you wake up than when you went to sleep.

I'm so sleepy when I wake up; I even end up napping throughout the day because I'm so tired.

This could be one of two things. One being any medications you are currently on. Some anti-depressants and anti-psychotics make you very tired; this holds true for many people. If it is not your medications, then it could be some form of sleep disorder that is making you not get enough quality sleep. Hypersomnia is where you feel excessive sleepiness during the day. You should speak with your doctor for further help.

I seem to have the exact opposite problem; I am not sleeping much at all.

Once again, this could be due to your medication interfering with your regular biological clock and wake/sleep cycles, or it could be something else. In any event, you would be best to check with your doctor as there may be something else at play. Something else to consider is if you have bipolar disorder, which is also known as manic depression, you might be in the middle of a manic episode where the need for sleep is greatly reduced.

Insights

Mental health and sleep are very closely related. Sleep deprivation has an alarming effect on our mental health and psychological state; moreover, people with mental health problems are more likely to have insomnia. However, according to several different studies, sleep problems often directly contribute to and increase the risk of psychiatric disorders, including depression and anxiety. For this reason, treating a sleep disorder may alleviate the symptoms of a simultaneously occurring mental health problem.

The Effect of Sleep on Mental Health

At present, there is not enough research to understand the basis of the mutual relationship between sleep and mental health. However, according to neurochemistry and neuroimaging studies, a good night's sleep helps make a person more emotionally and mentally resilient. In addition to this, chronic sleep deprivation is the most common cause of emotional vulnerability and negative thinking.

A healthy sleep cycle transitions between two significant categories every 90 minutes. A person progresses through four different stages of increasingly deep sleep during "quiet" sleep; breathing and heart rate slow down, muscles relax, and body temperature drops. Similarly, during the deepest stage of quiet sleep, physiological changes are produced, which help in boosting the functioning of the immune system.

The other category of sleep is rapid eye movement or REM sleep. REM sleep is the period during which people dream. It has been reported in studies that REM sleep contributes to emotional health, memory and learning in complex ways. During REM sleep, breathing, heart rate, blood pressure and body temperature increase to the same levels as when a person is awake. Sleep disruption, among other things, affects stress hormones and the levels of neurotransmitters; amplifying the effects of psychiatric disorders or vice versa.

The Link between Depression and Sleep

People diagnosed with depression often complain that they have trouble getting to sleep or staying asleep. The definitive link between lack of sleep and depression is the reason behind that. Moreover, one of the common signs of depression is an inability to fall asleep or insomnia. However, that does not mean that the primary cause of insomnia or any other sleep disorders is depression. Insomnia, at some point in life, affects nearly one out of three adults and is the most common sleep disorder in Australia. As people get older, insomnia becomes more prevalent. Likewise, compared to men, more women have insomnia. According to most experts, adults need seven to nine hours of sleep every night. However, the average Australian only gets 6.9 hours of sleep even without depression. Nonetheless, the problems of sleep are compounded when mixed with depression.

One of the critical signs of depression is an inability to sleep; another sign is either oversleeping or sleeping too much. Lack of sleep plays a role in depression; however, having a sleep disorder is not a cause of depression itself. Depression can be made worse because of a lack of sleep because of personal problems or other medical illnesses. An important clue that someone may be depressed is an inability to sleep that lasts over extended periods.

Although the figures differ slightly between studies undertaken, it is safe to say that over 70% of children and adolescents with depressive and/or psychiatric disorders suffer from sleep disturbances. This particular study also states that girls were more likely to have sleep disturbances than boys (77% vs 69.2%). As a whole, children with sleep disorders are more likely to suffer from more depressive symptoms vs children who do not have sleep disturbances. Of those children who were sleep disturbed, it was found that those who suffer from both insomnia and hypersomnia were even more susceptible to severe depressive episodes vs those who had only insomnia or hypersomnia alone.

When we consider how adults fare, estimates place 90 percent of patients with depression complain about sleep disturbances. In one particular study, of the 92% of study participants who reported sleep disturbances, 85.2% suffered from insomnia and 47.5% suffered from hypersomnia. It is noted that when both insomnia and hypersomnia are present in individuals, there was between a two- and three-fold increase in the risk of bipolar disorders[3]. Breathing disorders such as Obstructive Sleep Apnoea (OSA) are also prevalent amongst those who suffer from depression, with it being noted that the more severe the OSA is, the more likely depressive episodes are. Something interesting from this study was the conflicting assessment of effectiveness of treating OSA with regards to depression improvement. What is very clear, however, is that both OSA and depression should be treated together and not in isolation[4].

---

[3] Liu X, Buysse DJ, Gentzler AL, et al. Insomnia and hypersomnia associated with depressive phenomenology and comorbidity in childhood depression. *Sleep*. 2007;30(1):83-90. doi:10.1093/sleep/30.1.83

https://pubmed.ncbi.nlm.nih.gov/17310868/

[4] BaHammam AS, Kendzerska T, Gupta R, et al. Comorbid depression in obstructive sleep apnea: an under-recognized association. *Sleep Breath*. 2016;20(2):447-456. doi:10.1007/s11325-015-1223-x

https://pubmed.ncbi.nlm.nih.gov/26156890/

Insomnia and other sleep problems have a direct effect on the outcomes of patients with depression. Depressed patients who continue to be affected with depression, compared to those without sleep problems, are less likely to respond to treatment. Even patients showing improvement in antidepressant therapy, later on, are more at risk of relapse of depression[5].

There is also emerging evidence that patients who are suffering from sleep disturbances such as insomnia and hypersomnia are at more risk of suicidal behaviours including suicidal ideation, attempting suicide and ultimately death by suicide when compared to patients who regularly get a good night's sleep[6].

In some respects, sleep and mental health lifestyle changes are the recommended treatment for insomnia, the most common sleep problem. Also, regardless of a patient suffering from a psychiatric disorder, including depression, the treatment is similar for all patients of insomnia. The fundamentals of treatment include a combination of psychotherapy, behavioural strategies, lifestyle changes and drugs if necessary.

---

[5] Cutler AJ. The Role of Insomnia in Depression and Anxiety: Its Impact on Functioning, Treatment, and Outcomes. *J Clin Psychiatry.* 2016;77(8):e1010. doi:10.4088/JCP.14076tx3c

https://pubmed.ncbi.nlm.nih.gov/27561147/

[6] Bernert RA, Kim JS, Iwata NG, Perlis ML. Sleep disturbances as an evidence-based suicide risk factor. *Curr Psychiatry Rep.* 2015;17(3):554. doi:10.1007/s11920-015-0554-4

https://pubmed.ncbi.nlm.nih.gov/25698339/

Changes in Lifestyle

Most people know that caffeine, alcohol and nicotine contribute to sleeplessness. Initially, alcohol depresses the nervous system and helps some people fall asleep; however, as the effects wear off, people wake up after a few hours. Similarly, nicotine is a stimulant that speeds up the heart rate and thinking. Therefore, it is best to avoid these substances. If you cannot avoid them otherwise, then avoiding them before going to bed is another option.

Physical Activity

We have discussed exercise in another chapter already, but it's worth considering the benefits of physical activity and the relationship with better sleep.

Engaging in regular exercise helps contribute to a more restful sleep. Regular physical activity increases the time spent in deep sleep, which is the most physically and mentally restorative sleep phase. Deep sleep promotes better immune function, supports cardiac health and helps to control stress and anxiety.

Research also suggests that physical exercise can help with the severity of sleep disorders and may help reduce the symptoms of obstructive sleep apnoea.

I have been diagnosed in the past with obstructive sleep apnoea, and my wife tells me I used to snore like a thundercloud. I never heard it myself, but it must have been pretty bad. When I managed to lose some weight, things improved.

If you do have sleep apnoea, your doctor or physician will recommend getting a Continuous Positive Airway Pressure (CPAP) machine. The role of this machine is to keep your airways open during the night while you sleep thereby eliminating snoring and not feeling rested when you wake up in the morning.

Sleep Hygiene

There is a popular expert belief that people learn insomnia and can eventually learn to sleep better. The term "good sleep hygiene" is often used to include tips, for example, freeing yourself from distractions such as television or computer, using the bedroom only for sleeping, and maintaining a regular sleeping and waking schedule. Some experts also suggest staying awake longer to ensure that sleep is more restful.

Meditation

Meditation is an excellent way to reduce stress and anxiety – two of the prime candidates making it hard to go to sleep at night. In some instances, stress can make your existing sleep conditions even worse.

Meditation is a relaxation technique, which helps to alleviate stress and anxiety symptoms by promoting inner peace and helping quiet your mind and body collectively. When you meditate, several physiological changes occur in your mind and body. These may include:

- Increase of melatonin (a hormone which helps regulate your sleep and promote a better night's rest)
- An increase in serotonin (which is generally a precursor of melatonin, but which also helps with depression and other mental health disorders)
- Reducing your heart rate
- A decrease in blood pressure
- Activating parts of the brain that are responsible for controlling sleep.

Your body tends to experience the same sort of changes in the early stages of sleep, so as a direct result, meditation can help promote healthy sleep by initiating those changes.

So how do you meditate? I'm glad you asked!

The basic steps of meditation are as follows:

- Find yourself a quiet area of your home or wherever you are mediating. Sit or lie down, depending upon your personal preferences. Just a small tip: Lying down is preferable if it's bedtime.
- Close your eyes and breathe slowly and deeply. Inhale and exhale. Focus on your breathing.

- If any intrusive thoughts pop into your mind, let it go - refocus on your breathing to help with this.
- Remember that if it's your first time, only do between 3 and 5 minutes. It will take some time and practice before you get to the ideal period of between 15 and 20 minutes.

Cognitive Behavioural Therapy

Cognitive Behavioural Therapy for Insomnia (CBT-I) is an approved method for treating insomnia without the use of sleeping pills. Sounds a bit new, space-aged and hippy right? Well, it's a legitimate treatment and is used quite successfully with patients around the world. A recent scientific meeting concluded that CBT-I is an effective and safe means of managing chronic insomnia and its associated effects.[7]

Is its hard work? It sure can be. CBT-I aims to change the sleeping habits and any misconceptions around sleep and insomnia that help to perpetuate it.

CBT-I includes regular (probably weekly) visits to your doctor or physician, who will give you a series of sleep assessments and ask you to complete a sleep diary. They will then work with you in-depth to help change the way you are sleeping and provide feedback on the process.

---

[7] https://www.sleepfoundation.org/insomnia/treatment/cognitive-behavioral-therapy-insomnia

It's often reasonable to get less sleep than usual in the first few weeks, and sometimes you will need to practice a method called Sleep Restriction Therapy, which means no more napping in between your normal sleep cycle. You may also be told to not go to sleep until rather late in the evening. This is a normal part of CBT-I.

"You Know You're In Love When You Can't Fall
Asleep Because Reality Is Finally Better
Than Your Dreams."
– Dr Seuss

Summary

To summarise, we have spoken about the importance of sleep for both your physical and mental wellbeing. We discussed the potential link between sleep and depression. We then talked about sleep disorders before finally talking about ways to improve your sleep quality.

Action Plan

- If you are having sleeping problems, make sure you see your GP about it.
- Keep a sleep diary to help record your sleeping patterns.
- Be aware that some medications can make you very tired.
- Sleep disorders can interfere with your natural sleep cycle.

CHAPTER 7

The Power of a Positive Mind

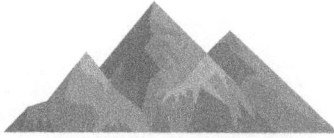

"We cannot solve our problems with the same thinking we used to create them."

– Albert Einstein

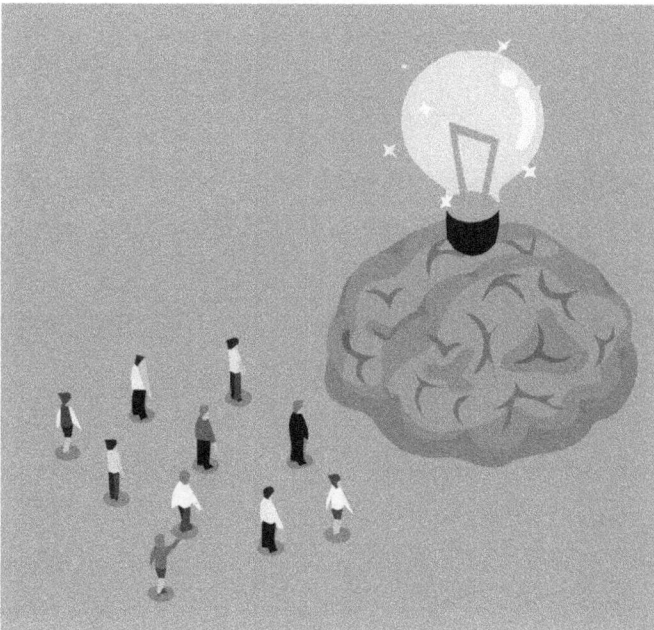

COMMON THOUGHTS

I just cannot concentrate on anything anymore!

Often, I've thought those same words. Some days it's utterly impossible to concentrate on anything. But what I have found is that if you set yourself a tiny goal, even something as simple as having a shower, once you have completed it, you have accomplished something, and hopefully you will be more comfortable to continue achieving goals for the day.

My relationship has fallen apart, and now I'm completely lost.

It's ok to feel that way after a relationship ends. Nobody expects you to be bright and bubbly straight away. Make sure you take some time for yourself and practise self-care whenever possible. Spend time with friends and family, live life. Gradually things will get easier for you.

There is nothing positive in my life; how do you expect me to find something positive!

Well, while it might be challenging to find something positive, look for something simple. What about the love of your family? Or your partner/spouse? Your pet? Anything at all.

Insights

Having a positive mindset can help your depression immensely. I found this out the hard way for many years. I would always imagine the worst probable outcome for any given scenario, and then it would happen. I didn't even give myself a fighting chance! While I'm not a huge believer in putting it out there, I have found that often if you don't expect the worst to happen, it doesn't happen.

I have a golden rule that I always apply, which is never put two depressed people in the same room at the same time. It's a bit tongue in cheek, but what I'm saying is being around other people who are thinking negatively will rub off on you no matter how hard you try. So, if you're feeling down and in a depressive headspace, try to surround yourself with positive people.

Depression is a battle between your mind and you. So, if you can, try and read some self-development books or watch videos of people from the self-development space. Good ones you can check out are Tony Robbins, Gary Vaynerchuk; even Arnold Schwarzenegger is quite inspirational. Check out YouTube or Facebook; both are great places to look at videos.

Goal Setting

When you are suffering from a mental health illness, you may find that your productivity is decreased or even non-existent. The ability to complete even the smallest task becomes a real challenge. I will occasionally have those sorts of days and sometimes even weeks. I used to get angry and annoyed with myself; in fact, I still do but not as much as I used to.

Try setting yourself small but achievable goals on a daily basis. At the end of the day, if you have gotten through your list, congratulations are in order. If you didn't get through your list, make sure you acknowledge what you did get accomplished and be happy.

Goal setting was super crucial for me while I was trekking the Inca Trail in Peru. Having small but well-defined goals made it possible for me to complete the Inca Trail.

My main goal for each day was simply to reach camp. On the fourth day, my goal was to reach the Sun Gates at Machu Picchu. Oh, and there was one more goal for the fourth day, which I didn't know about until it was upon me. The ultimate goal of climbing "The Gringo Killer Stairs".

But that's not the only time I set myself goals. Writing this book is another example. I didn't just sit down and write it from cover to cover all in one hit. I would set myself a goal of spending 25-30 minutes every few days to continue fleshing out the chapters.

When I was satisfied with the section, I would move on and start the next one. Sometimes I would get stuck or wasn't sure what I wanted to say so I would move onto the next and come back, later on, to work on it more.

Try looking at your daily activities and setting yourself small and realistic goals to complete. Think of them like manageable chunks of time. Maybe it's something as simple as getting out of bed at a predefined time of the morning. Or it could be doing some work for a specified period.

I recently watched an interesting video of a US Navy Admiral speaking at university graduation. He said, if you want to change the world, start by making your bed every morning. Ok, you might be thinking WTF - what does that have to do with anything? The logic is that by making your bed in the morning, you have completed your first goal for the day, and it will be easier to achieve the next goal and so on. If you would like to watch the video presentation, you will find it under my YouTube Channel under the Motivational Videos Playlist.

This next tip came from my psychologist. He said it helps to look forward to certain activities like going on holidays. You should try and plan something every three to six months if possible, which you can look forward to. It doesn't have to be anything massive, even going away for the weekend is excellent for you.

The Two Minds Syndrome

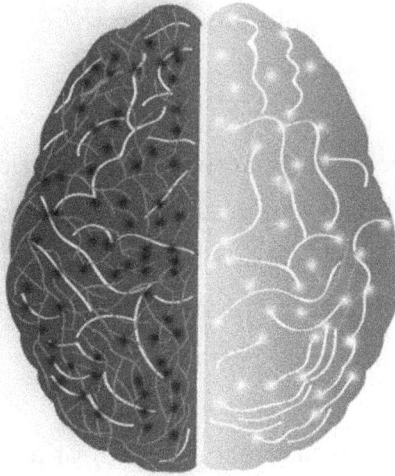

I am a firm believer that everyone has a "default" mode when it comes to mindset and thinking. It might be that you are naturally a negative thinker, or you might be a usually positive thinker. Heck, you might just sit smack bang in the middle of both. I personally call this the "Two Minds Syndrome," indicating both positive and negative thinking.

In numerous cultures, the ages between 5 and 7 are recognised as the start of the "age of reason". So, between the ages of 6 and 12 are generally regarded as exceptionally important in the development of children. It is not uncommon for chores or tasks to be assigned to kids to help promote a healthy understanding of responsibility without jeopardising the ability to still be a child[8].

---

[8] Collins, W. A., & National Research Council. (1984). Cognitive Development In School-Age Children: Conclusions And New Directions. In Development During Middle Childhood: The Years From Six to Twelve. National Academies Press (US). https://www.ncbi.nlm.nih.gov/books/NBK216770/

In another study, a group of mothers were interviewed about what age range they considered to have the most parental influence, that is being able to effectively guide their adolescents towards the "perceived" right path. Somewhat surprisingly, 78% of mothers nominated the age range of 10 and above, with a very strong preference towards the age ranges of 10 and 15 years old[9].

As you can see from the studies that have been undertaken, between the ages of 6 and up to 15 years old are going to be the years that drastically shape how you perceive the world, the way in which you cope with changes and how you think. I also happen to think it's not just your parents and immediate family who will help shape you, but also close friends and acquaintances. Real-world experiences are also going to count immensely in this as well, not only the experiences but how you chose to deal with those experiences.

From what my parents have told me of my childhood and my own memories, it was a pretty happy time for me and would have been generally positive. I'm relatively sure however I know where the wheels fell off for me. It was the death of my grandfather when I was 12 years old; it seems that was a critical defining moment of my life, and it helped shape me to be a negative thinker. The death of a loved one is never an easy thing to deal with, as I found out.

Sometimes I wish I could go back and give my younger self a bit of a pep talk and help guide him towards a more positive mindset,

[9] Worthman, C. M., Tomlinson, M., & Rotheram-Borus, M. J. (2016). When can parents most influence their child's development? Expert knowledge and perceived local realities. Social Science & Medicine, 154, 62-69.
https://www.ncbi.nlm.nih.gov/pmc/articles/PMC4826572/

but then that wouldn't be me, and my life would probably have been drastically different to what it is now. I should have been concentrating on all the great memories of my grandfather, and not the overwhelming sadness of not having him around anymore. This is something I have spoken to my own children about, that while it's ok the be sad and to miss the person who is gone – we shouldn't forget all the great times we had with them as that should be their legacy.

It seems like as a society in general we do not really discuss the subject of death until it happens to somebody we know, like a family member or close relative/friend. We really need to discuss this subject a little more than we do – not to scare our children but to let them know that it is a normal part of life.

I would like to think I handle the death of family members and loved ones far better than I used to. I'm still sad and upset, of course, but I now try and remember all the good times with that person.

My maternal grandmother passed away in the middle of 2018. She was diagnosed with Multiple Sclerosis when she was younger, but she never let it stop her from living her life. It was only in the last five to ten years she had to use a wheelchair to get around. I remember sitting on the back veranda facing the waterfront and chatting with Grandma for hours on end. Those are the memories that I choose to remember and not my last memories of her which were her very sick and frail and in hospital.

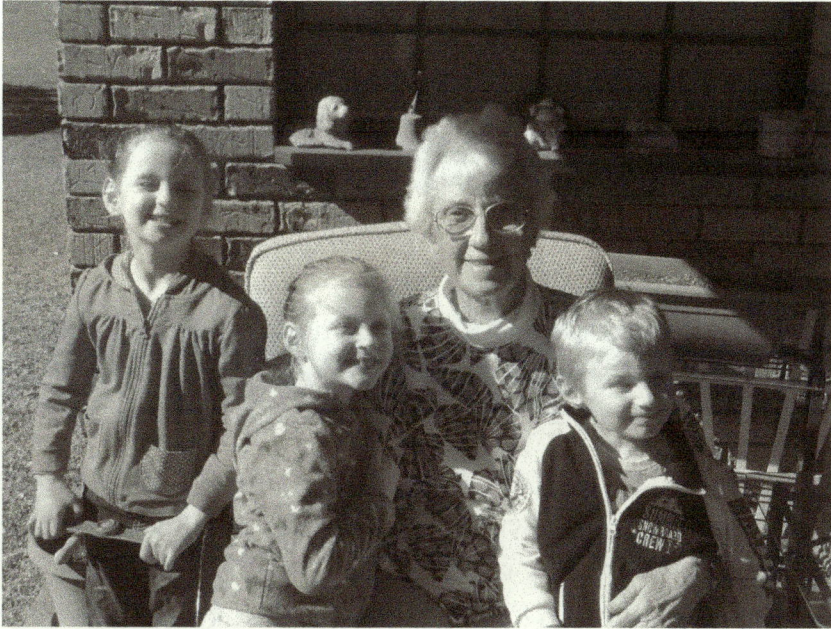

Grandma and Chelsea, Jasmine and Zachery

Of course, I'm not suggesting that you can simply erase X amount of years' worth of negative thinking overnight - it's going to take some time and practice. Even I still battle on occasion with negative thoughts. Sometimes a situation just does not have a silver lining, and if that's the case, then don't beat yourself up about thinking negatively. Just do not let it stop you from pursuing positive thoughts where you can and continuing to live your life

Gratitude

Recently I've noticed on social media a lot of people stating that telling somebody who is depressed to 'practise gratitude' isn't going to help them at all. I tend to disagree with that statement. It's not so much that practising gratitude is going to fix your mental health illness, but it does provide an interesting opportunity for you. Let's say you have had a couple of negative events happen in your day, and you have been keeping track of some of the good things that have happened to you on the same day, practising gratitude can help provide perspective that the whole day wasn't a complete write-off. Remember, this is a battle between your mind and you – the more ammunition you have to help show your mind it wasn't so bad, the better you're likely to feel.

So, you might be asking yourself, how do I practise gratitude? Let me share some ideas with you.

- Tell someone you love them and how much you appreciate them – this could be your spouse/partner/family members.
- Notice the beauty in nature each day – you could go for a bushwalk or a stroll along the beach.
- Spend time working on your friendships – great friendships take work and commitment.
- Smile more often – something so simple, can be so powerful.
- Watch some motivational movies on YouTube or Facebook – there are some excellent videos out there.
- There are so many different ways to practise gratitude – try a Google search to look at all the different methods.

Keeping a gratitude diary is also a great idea. You record the things for which you are grateful for daily, and when your mood is not as good as you would like, you can revisit the diary and read the things that you have been thankful for recently.

"Don't Be Pushed Around by The Fears in Your Mind.
Be Led by The Dreams in Your Heart."
– Roy T. Bennett

Summary

We talked about how the people you hang out with can help forge your new positive mindset or collectively drag you down into negative thinking. We spoke about watching some motivational movies on YouTube or Facebook - often these will help build you up. We talked about goal setting and why it's so important. We also spoke about how you should make these goals realistic, so you're not setting yourself up for failure in the beginning. We talked about the two-minds syndrome, and how everyone seems to have a default thinking mode which oftentimes has been learned during our critical years of growing (6 to 15 years old). We also spoke about gratitude and how practising daily gratitude can help to improve your mental wellbeing.

Action Plan

- Set some simple goals for yourself.
- Don't be down on yourself if you don't finish all of your goals for a single day. Just getting one done is an achievement in itself.
- Determine if you are a positive or negative thinker and work on aiming for positive thoughts.
- Visit my YouTube Channel and view the Motivational Playlist.

CHAPTER 8

Breaking Out of Your Mind Prison

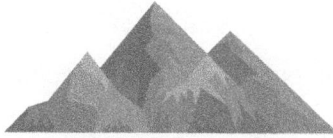

"I don't care what you think unless it is about me."
– Kurt Cobain

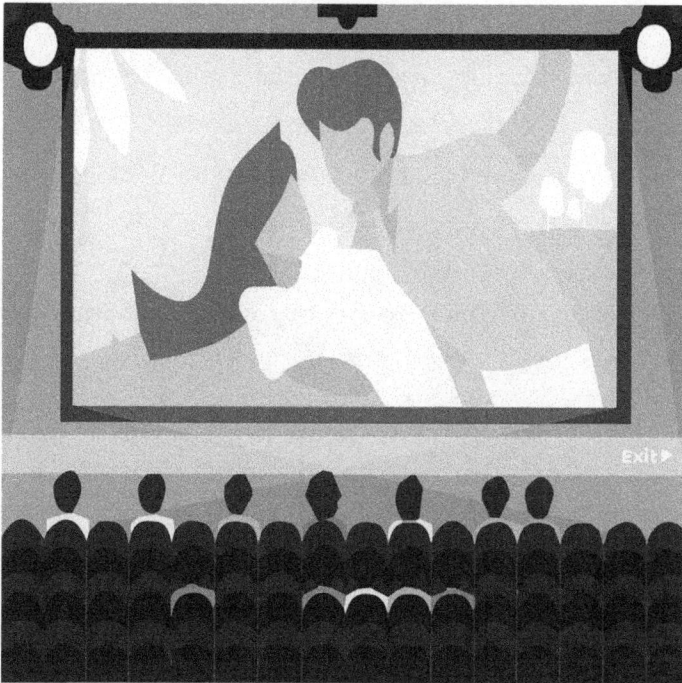

COMMON THOUGHTS

I promised my friend I would come to their party, but I don't want to go.

Firstly, take a deep breath and calm yourself. You have got this, and you can do it. Now, why don't you want to go to the party? Is it because you're afraid of what others will think of you? Why should you care what anybody thinks of you, just be happy to be you. If you dislike it so much, leave.

But what if people think I'm a loser?

Well, you can't control what others will think about you - that's one of the first things to remember. And be 100% honest with yourself, does it matter if they believe you are a loser? It's just their opinion.

I have trouble just doing my grocery shopping, what can I do?

The struggle is real, and you have taken the first step in getting help for your extreme anxiety. Medication might help you as well as seeing a psychologist regularly. Remember above all else to be kind to yourself, because if you won't be kind, why would others?

Insights

Isolation and loneliness can be a big part of people's lives when they have a mental illness, whether it be depression or anxiety or even schizophrenia. Your illness makes you feel less and less like being social, and you start to isolate yourself from both your friends and family.

Almost one-third of Australians surveyed who have psychotic disorders are living alone, and of that figure, 39% of these people do not have a "best friend" who they can share their thoughts and feelings with.

You might isolate yourself because you think you are a burden on your friends and family. You might isolate yourself because you just don't want to have to talk to anyone. There might be a heap of reasons, and I can't list them all here because I don't know them all. Everybody is so unique and different and has their reasons for what they do and how they do it.

There is also the issue of the associated stigma with mental health illnesses and the disadvantage and social exclusion that people with mental illness can face. And it doesn't matter if you are living with somebody or not; it affects both groups equally.

Social Distancing, Self-Isolation and COVID-19

You would have to be living under a rock to have not heard about COVID-19, also known as coronavirus. It busted down the doors in January of 2020, the likes of which we haven't seen before in modern times, and we are still dealing with the fallout from this viral illness.

Many countries implemented strict lockdown rules to help prevent the spread of this deadly virus. Two laws in particular, in place in Australia and other countries - social distancing and self-isolation – will cause some issues for those both with and without mental health illnesses. It's a generally accepted view that those who are extroverted tend to thrive around other people and get their energy from being social while those who are introverted tend to rely on themselves and draw their energy from being alone. Most people will categorise themselves as either being "introverted" or "extroverted". The reality is somewhat more intriguing than you might at first think.

The terms "introvert" and "extrovert" were popularised by a man called Carl G. Jung in the early 20th century. It seems between then and now the meanings of those terms got confused by society and we started to accept that every person either fit into one term or the other. However, what Carl really meant was that these two terms represented the very extreme ends of a scale. So really, most of us would actually be somewhere between these two extremes on the scale.

"There is no such thing as a pure introvert or
extrovert. Such a person would be in
the lunatic asylum."
– Carl G. Jung

Ambivert Personality Continuum Scale

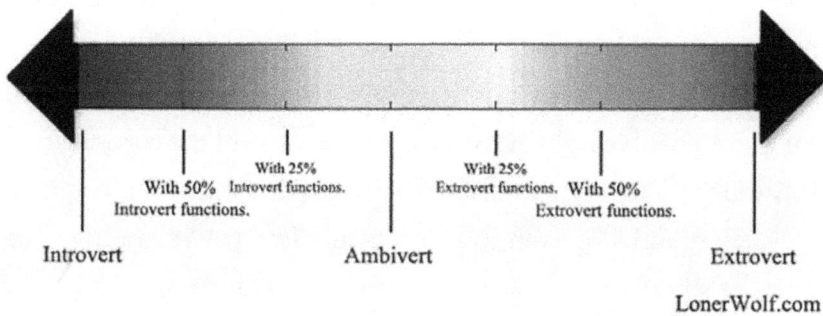

With 25%
Introvert functions.

With 50%
Introvert functions.

With 25%
Extrovert functions.

With 50%
Extrovert functions.

Introvert   Ambivert   Extrovert

LonerWolf.com

Source[10]

As we know from having a mental illness and that I can certainly attest to, we tend to withdraw from society and social settings as they cause us too much trouble and make it harder for us to manage our emotions. So we would fit more within the Introvert and Ambivert portion of the above scale. It has been joked about on Facebook that those of us who are more introverted have been training for this all our lives.

Before researching this topic while writing this book, I often thought that I was simply "Introverted" and that was it. Now,

---

[10] https://commons.wikimedia.org/wiki/File:Ambivert_personality_continu-um_scale.png

I recognise that I probably fit neatly between the Introvert and Extrovert scale and identify as Ambivert. While I am more than happy to sit back and be alone and enjoy my own company, when the situation calls for it, I can also be a social person and will happily interact with others, once I have built up my courage a little and worked past some of my anxieties.

When you have a mental illness, you already feel isolated and alone, and the advice given usually is to try and socialise a bit, meet up with friends and family and generally try to get out a bit. Well, that is not possible right at the moment because of the coronavirus. How long will this be the case? Honestly, I don't know; it could be for a few months or even longer. By the time you're reading this book, let's pray that the worst is over and behind us.

But what about those who would identify more between the Ambivert and Extrovert portion of the above scale? What sort of impact is the current pandemic crisis going to have on these sorts of people? Quite honestly, I feel it will be just as frustrating and dangerous for them as it is for those of us who have mental illnesses. We know that these types of people thrive and in general require more social interaction and that they "recharge their batteries" by this type of activity.

However, the imposed social distancing and self-isolation on us all by our governments is likely to cause many issues regarding mental health, both new cases and existing alike. It is quite possible, and dare I say more than likely that this current pandemic crisis will fuel another crisis, in the mental health arena this time.

Right now and more than ever, you need to identify ways you can stay connected with friends and family. You could video call your friends and family using Facetime, Skype, etc. You can interact with your friends and family using social media such as Facebook and Instagram. If you live alone and you are up for the responsibility, you can get yourself a pet cat, dog, bird or fish to help keep you company. I have three cats, so that helps to keep me company when I'm not feeling the best. Do keep in mind that pets are for life, so don't go down this route if you're not in it for the long haul as it's not fair to the animals.

Make sure you stay connected with your health professionals, some may offer Telehealth services while others will continue to offer face-to-face consultations and even a combination of both where the situation calls for it.

On a more personal note, while I would like to say that my mental health has not deteriorated throughout this period of uncertainty, it would be a lie. Living in Melbourne, Australia, we have been subjected to some of the harshest public health orders that I am aware of from around the world. I wanted to add this into the book here to illustrate that it doesn't matter how "together" you have your life – it can still rear its ugly head at times and cause issues. Remember to be kind to yourself during these times, and also kind and compassionate to others. You really never do know what somebody else is going through.

Co-dependency

Co-dependency is when the person requires another for their emotional, physical and social wellbeing. Co-dependent people attach their sense of self-worth to the approval of another. These people will struggle to function in the real world due to their unhealthy expectations. Some of the symptoms of co-dependency include persistent efforts to please others, poor boundaries and constant obsession about things that other people are doing all the time.

Most people grow up in a loving and nurturing environment, where we learn the required skills to function independently and create our sense of self-worth. Those with co-dependency typically grow up in a household that is lacking in that nurturing environment. It's marked by silence, unrealistic expectations and shaming.

Frequently co-dependency can make depression and other mental health illnesses worse as they will not acknowledge their own needs and desires. If you are living in a co-dependent relationship, you need to look into getting help as it is not healthy for either person.

Anxiety

Throughout the book, we have discussed depression and other mental health illnesses, but I thought it time to discuss anxiety. Anxiety can often be a very debilitating illness.

Anxiety is a set of responses the body creates to a given situation and prepares the body for the flight-or-fight response. It used to be perfect back when we were hunters and gatherers, but not so much anymore.

How it works is the brain will perceive danger or threat by any of the five senses which will send a signal to the nervous system, which will then trigger a release of adrenaline into your bloodstream. It is this secretion of adrenaline which helps make a person more alert and ready to execute the flight-or-fight response.

Some of the symptoms you may get when you have anxiety are as follows:

- Physical Symptoms
    - Rapid heartbeat
    - Difficulty breathing
    - Chest pain
    - Sweating
    - Dizziness
    - Numbness in toes, fingers and other extremities
    - Nausea
    - Exhaustion
    - Muscle tension
    - Shaking
    - Change in body temperature
    - Vision disturbances
- Cognitive Symptoms
    - Worry

- o Negative thinking
- o Difficulty in concentrating and attention
- Behavioural Symptoms
  - o Avoiding places, situations, people, objects and even memories
  - o Protective behaviours
  - o Aggressive attitude

Your doctor will diagnose you with anxiety after doing a complete physical examination, which helps to rule out other reasons for those symptoms. This is an important step, as some medical conditions have the same or similar symptoms, and your doctor doesn't want to miss those. Your doctor may also administer a simple questionnaire which helps rate the severity of your anxiety. Treatment options for anxiety include psychotherapy and medication primarily (similar to how depression is treated). The length of treatment varies between patient to patient, so it's not possible to predict how long it will take to manage your anxiety. It could be a short three- to six-month stint, or it could be much longer.

As I mentioned, I also suffer from anxiety, but it's not as bad as it used to be. When I was younger, and at school, my body used to get so worked up that I would blackout for some time. Luckily, it never happened anywhere that could cause a problem.

Now I still get anxiety, but it seems to be centred around unfamiliar activities. As an example, I'm happy to drive in really heavy traffic but only as long as I know exactly where

I'm going and what lane I should be in at that point. Otherwise, I'm a complete and utter nervous wreck. With the advent of GPS and map technologies on our phones, I've improved, but I still get somewhat nervous when I have to go somewhere new. I also have a bit of social anxiety when I'm out in gatherings and meeting new people. Once I have gotten to know them, it's much better, and I don't have the issue. The other weird time I get anxiety is when I'm cooking a new recipe. For some reason, not knowing all the steps upfront makes me a bit of a nervous wreck when cooking.

Strategies to Relax or Distract

Over the years, I have used several different methods to relax or distract me. Particularly with the schizoaffective disorder, sometimes I've needed to distract myself. Let me go into some of them for you.

- Listening to music is a relaxing and distracting mechanism for me. I've noticed the type of music playing can have a significant effect on my mood. If the song is happy or upbeat, it raises my spirits. A sad song will generally will bring me down.
- Playing computer games is another relaxing and distracting method for me. I'm a fan of retro games, so I often play games from my childhood/teenage years. But I also like the more modern games such as StarCraft II, Diablo III or even World of Warcraft.

- Reading a good book. I've always been a pretty avid reader, so I enjoy reading a good book. I'm one of those people who can re-read the same series over and over and over again. My favourite authors are David Eddings, Stephen King, Dean Koontz and Robert Jordan.

- Watching a movie is also a good distraction for me. Depending on the genre of film I'm watching it can help increase or decrease moods for me. My favourite film styles are horror, sci-fi, fantasy, and action. My current favourite movies are the new IT movies (Chapter 1 and 2) however I'm also a fan of the Star Wars movies - all nine of them.

- I'm a fan of water, so I find going for a walk along the beach at night-time is especially relaxing for me. Walking at the water's edge, and the moon out and shining bright is simply magical.

- Doing some exercise - I find exercise to be very therapeutic, as I can often walk and think at the same time. I find my mind to be very active and agile so I can think of all sorts of things when I'm walking.

Tips to Beat Isolation and Loneliness

Here are some tips for beating the isolation and loneliness. I've used a number of these methods over the years to help.

- Pet ownership - Pets are fantastic and can help during periods of stress, ill-health or isolation. Pets make excellent companions.

- Volunteering - When you are helping others, it helps to make you feel more connected.
- Friends and family - Being in contact with loved ones help to prevent isolation and loneliness. And just because family don't live near you, don't think you are out of luck. Remember that technology helps to keep us connected with those we love.
- Regular outings - When you have a mental illness, you won't generally feel like socialising, but try making an effort to get out and about with friends and family. Even doing the shopping can be a regular outing.
- Hobbies or learning - You can try a new hobby or even take up an old one. Learning a new skill or enrolling to study can also be a great way to help break through the isolation.
- Remember to look after yourself - make sure you keep up with your hygiene and eat proper meals. You should also make sure you get some exercise.

"If You Want to Conquer the Anxiety of Life,
Live in The Moment, Live in The Breath."
– Amit Ray

Summary

We spoke about how having a mental illness can make you feel isolated and lonely. There is still a stigma associated with mental illness (not as bad as it used to be, but it still does exist).

We talked about COVID-19 and how it has affected us. We spoke about co-dependency and how it's not beneficial for you, as either the co-dependent or the other person. We talked about anxiety, how is it diagnosed, treated, and how long it might take to get better and complete treatment. We talked about strategies to help relax and distract you when you are in the middle of a crisis (it doesn't matter if its anxiety, depression or schizophrenia – these methods should work equally well). And finally, we discussed some tips for beating isolation and loneliness.

Action Plan

- Speak to your doctor if you are worried about anxiety or you think that it plays a big part in your life.
- You might need to take medications and undertake psychotherapy – so don't be worried about either of these things.
- Identify which relaxation and distraction techniques work for you and make a note of them in case you need them in a hurry, or somebody else does.
- Try and implement some of the tips to help beat isolation and loneliness.

Afterword

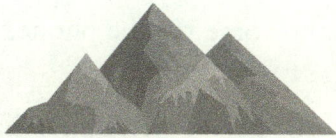

Congratulations on reaching the end of my book. By now I hope that you can see that just because you have a mental illness, it doesn't have to define your life and control you. So many people in the world suffer from mental health illnesses, and a large amount of research and studies that are being done on a near-constant basis should give you hope for a better future.

I want nothing more than for you to be able to manage your mental illness, whether that be depression, anxiety, bipolar or schizophrenia. I'm living proof because you can do it, and there are ways forward always.

I've noticed over the last few years that you are going to have great days, and then you are going to have some crappy days. It's just part and parcel of living with a mental illness. Don't be too hard on yourself; I always say a new day brings a fresh perspective and hopefully will get you back on track.

If you're anything like me, I always seem to have a crisis in the evenings and weekends when a lot of support workers and mental health practitioners are not available. And if they are available, you need to go into the local hospital to try and access those services. Which generally means hours upon hours of waiting. If you're suicidal, you should call the emergency services, 000 in Australia, 911 in the USA, or 999 in UK. Otherwise, you can look up mental health services on the internet – some offer web-based chat services and some via the phone.

You can visit my website at www.craigmarchant.com for further resources and information. I try and keep as much up to date news on my website as I can. If you are interested in speaking with me via Zoom or good old phone, then you can visit my website and drop me an enquiry.

About the Author

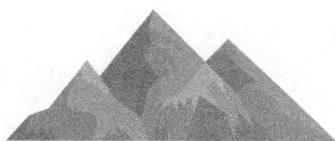

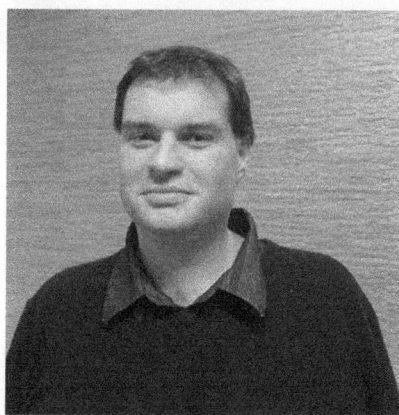

Craig Marchant has one mission which is to show others who suffer from mental health disorders that they can live a great life. Craig says, "Having a mental illness does not have to be a death sentence, and you can become the best version of yourself if you set your mind to it."

After completing the Inca Trail in 2016, which raised funds for the Leukaemia Foundation here in Australia, and then returning to work, Craig discovered his passion for helping others. He decided to leave the businesses he helped build and set out to help other people improve their mental health and quality of life.

Craig says, "Trekking the Inca Trail in Peru was just what I needed. It showed me that I was so much stronger than I gave myself credit for and that I could do anything that I set my mind to."

Craig believes this challenge was a game-changer for him and now wants to help others realise their full potential and undertake their own physical challenge.

Craig is the eldest child of Peter and Kathy, brother to Mathew and Angela, husband to Kendyl and devoted father of five children, Chelsea, Jasmine, Zachery, Aidyn and Jace. Craig lives with his wife and kids in Narre Warren South, VIC, Australia.

If you would like to reach out and speak to Craig, you can find his details below:

Website:	https://www.craigmarchant.com/
Email:	info@craigmarchant.com
Facebook Profile:	https://www.facebook.com/craig.marchant.7758
Facebook Page:	https://www.facebook.com/craigmarchant81/
Facebook Group:	https://www.facebook.com/groups/mental.health.demystified

Acknowledgments

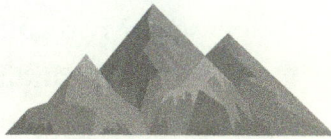

There are several people who I would like to acknowledge.

Firstly, I would like to thank my mum and dad. They put up with so much from us kids, and not only that; I must have cost them a small fortune in my education, especially with all the courses and seminars I attended over the years while still at school. For the countless hours spent with me at doctors' appointments, hospitals, and everything in between. And most importantly, for never giving up on me, even when I was ready to give up on myself.

Next, thank you to all the doctors, nurses, psychologists, and psychiatrists over the years who have helped me. I more than likely would not be here today without all of them. It is sometimes quite a thankless job, so here is my chance to say thank you for everything that you do

I would like to especially mention my current psychologist and the author of the foreword in my book, Dr John Di Battista. I have known John now for several years, and he has helped me through some major events in my life. I always say your psychologist should be both knowledgeable and empathetic, as without either of those important skills, it is difficult to form a professional bond.

I would like to thank Speakers Institute for showing me that I have a voice, and how I can use it. My thanks especially to Sam and Kate Cawthorn for helping and guiding me in the right direction, and more importantly for not letting me give up on myself when it would have been all too easy.

To the wonderful members and leaders of Speakers Tribe and especially Speakers Tribe Victoria. I am honoured to be part of such an amazing group and to benefit from all the combined wisdom and knowledge contained within.

To Natasa, Stuart, and the whole team at Ultimate 48 Hour Author – thank you for making the process to get my book completed and published a lot easier than I ever imagined it could be. Your guidance and support have been outstanding, and I would not have wanted to do it without you all.

Lastly, but certainly not least I would like to thank my business coach Kaylene Ledgar. Kaylene also doubles as my therapist, sounding board, and generally helps me out far more than she may realise. Her guidance, support and encouragement have been invaluable to me.

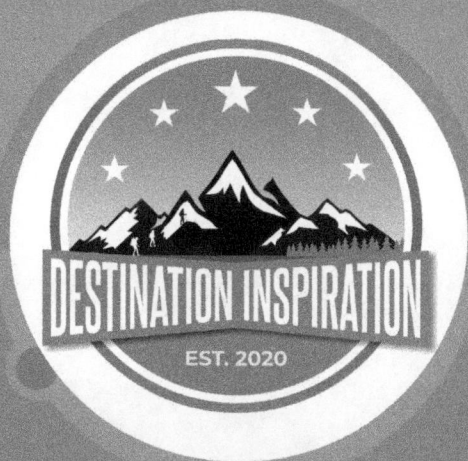

CRAIG
M A R C H A N T

DESTINATION INSPIRATION
EST. 2020

Undertaking the physical challenge of the Inca Trail in Peru on behalf of the Leukaemia Foundation and raising funds for research and support of those who suffer from blood cancer was one of the most pivotal moments in my life.

To be able to support such a worthwhile charity while going on a journey of self-discovery was a truly inspirational adventure, one which will stay with me for the rest of my life.

But it got me thinking, would others who suffer from mental health illnesses also be able to benefit from such an adventure? it is with that thought that I have devised an innovative and exciting opportunity for those who have mental health issues to better learn about themselves.

Thus, Destination Inspiration was born. A business dedicated to helping you to achieve your own success, and help you see that you do not have to let your mental illness define you, you can define it.

We will travel to inspiring and exciting destinations such as:

- The Larapinta Trail in the Northern Territory, Australia

- The Inca Trail in Peru

- And many more.

The program will provide you with both pre and post support sessions, to help you make the most out of your life-changing adventure. We will also handle all of your flight and accommodation requirements, along with most meals. Experienced guides will be on hand to help us on our journey and team leaders with who you can discuss and talk about anything. We will also donate to one of the many wonderful mental health charities here in Australia, so that your own journey of self-discovery can help others in need as well.

Ready for the adventure of your life with amazing supportive resources.

Register your interest here by visiting
www.craigmarchant.com/destination-inspiration
for more details and to sign up to our waiting list – ready for when
we launch our first adventure.

181

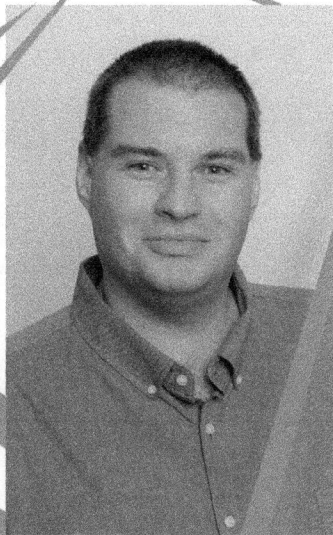

CRAIG MARCHANT

For some people suffering from a mental illness, just waking up and going about their daily lives can be a considerable challenge. Let alone to dream of Trekking the Ancient Inca Trail in Peru.

But for Craig Marchant, this awe-inspiring dream became a reality and with it, a newfound passion which helped ignite his personal goal of helping those who suffer mental illness to live a fulfilling life.

As a seasoned business entrepreneur in the Information Technology sector, including as the Chief Technical Officer for one of Australia's fastest-growing web hosting and domain name businesses, Craig has a unique understanding of what it takes to succeed.

Being diagnosed with Depression, Anxiety and Schizoaffective Disorder at a young age, Craig has had to learn how to manage his illnesses while getting on with life. Navigating life and all the challenges and hurdles it presents is no easy feat.

Craig has three signature keynotes that he can deliver to your audience, whether that be a small or large group and depending on your requirements. These keynotes are:

- **Conquer Your Inner Demons – One Man's Journey On The Path To Self-Discovery**

  Key takeaways from this keynote:

  - o Challenging yourself and stepping out of your comfort zone can promote better self-awareness and improve your mental state
  - o Having a mental illness does not have to define you, you can define it
  - o Following your dreams can be scary, but so very worthwhile.

- **Keeping It In The Family – A Father's Perspective On Mental Health Illnesses In Children**

  Key takeaways from this keynote:

  - o Don't blame yourself, the reasons for mental illness are very complex
  - o Understanding how you can help your child with their illness and recovery
  - o Promoting trust between your child and yourself is essential to their well-being and recovery.

- **See The Person Beneath – Schizophrenia and Schizoaffective Disorder Are Mental Illnesses as Well**

  Key takeaways from this keynote:

  - o Why those who suffer from Schizophrenia / Schizoaffective Disorder and other related illnesses feel abandoned and alone
  - o Practical ways you can help somebody who suffers from these conditions
  - o The person beneath the illness is still just a human being, longing to be accepted and understood.

Craig is also able to create a custom message to deliver to your audience based around mental health topics such as Depression, Anxiety, Schizophrenia / Schizoaffective Disorder and Suicide / Suicide Prevention.

Craig travels from Melbourne, Australia and is happy to speak and consult across the world.

+61 432 408 897   info@craigmarchant.com   www.craigmarchant.com

183

www.ingramcontent.com/pod-product-compliance
Lightning Source LLC
Chambersburg PA
CBHW031125020426
42333CB00012B/230